Inflammatory Bowel Disease
Experience and Controversy

A Teaching Seminar on Inflammatory Bowel Disease
Sponsored by Lenox Hill Hospital (New York)
and the American College of Gastroenterology

Edited by

BURTON I. KORELITZ, MD

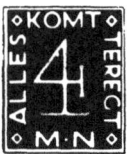

1982
MARTINUS NIJHOFF PUBLISHERS
THE HAGUE / BOSTON / LONDON

Library of Congress Cataloging in Publication Data
Teaching Seminar on Inflammatory Bowel Disease
    (1979) : Lenox Hill Hospital)
    Inflammatory bowel disease.

    Bibliography: p.
    Includes index.
    1. Enteritis--Congresses. 2. Enteritis, Regional--Congresses. I. Korelitz, Burton I.,
1926-   . II. Lenox Hill Hospital. III. American College of Gastroenterology. IV. Title.
(DNLM: 1. Intestinal diseases--Congresses. 2. Inflammation –Congresses. 3. Crohn
disease--Congresses.   WI 420 T253i 1979]
RC862.E5T42   1979   616.3'44   81-4954
ISBN-13: 978-94-009-7441-8   e-ISBN-13: 978-94-009-7439-5
DOI: 10.1007/978-94-009-7439-5   AACR2

Distributors for all countries outside North America

Kluwer Academic Publishers Group
Distribution Center
P.O. Box 322
3300 AH Dordrecht
The Netherlands

Joint edition published by

MARTINUS NIJHOFF PUBLISHERS
P.O. Box 566, 2501 CN The Hague, The Netherlands
and
John Wright • PSG Inc
545 Great Road
Littleton, Massachusetts 01460, U.S.A.

This volume is listed in the Library of Congress Cataloging in Publication Data

ISBN-13: 978-94-009-7441-8

CONTRIBUTORS

Arthur H. Aufses, Jr, MD
Chairman and Franz W. Sichel
  Professor
Department of Surgery
Mount Sinai School of Medicine
  of the City University of New York
New York, New York

Theodore M. Bayless, MD
Associate Professor of Medicine
The Johns Hopkins University School
  of Medicine,
Physician
The Johns Hopkins Hospital
Baltimore, Maryland

Michael S. Bruno, MD
Director of Medicine
Lenox Hill Hospital, and
Professor of Medicine and
  Associate Dean
New York Medical College
New York, New York

Robert S. Coles, MD
Director of Ophthalmology
Lenox Hill Hospital, and
Associate Clinical Professor of
  Ophthalmology
Mount Sinai School of Medicine of the
  City University of New York
New York, New York

Richard G. Farmer, MD
Chairman, Department of Medicine
Director, Division of
  Gastroenterology
Cleveland Clinic
Cleveland, Ohio

Harry D. Fein, MD
Consulting Physician
Formerly Chief of Gastroenterology
Lenox Hill Hospital, and
Associate Professor of Clinical
  Medicine
New York University School of
  Medicine
New York, New York

Irwin Gelernt, MD
Associate Clinical Professor
Department of Surgery
Mount Sinai School of Medicine of the
City University of New York
New York, New York

Myron D. Goldberg, MD
Assistant Adjunct Physician
  (Gastroenterology)
Lenox Hill Hospital
New York, New York

Mansho T. Khilnani, MD
Consulting Radiologist
Lenox Hill Hospital, and
Clinical Professor of Radiology
Mount Sinai School of Medicine of the
City University of New York
New York, New York

Burton I. Korelitz, MD
Chief of Gastroenterology
Lenox Hill Hospital, and
Clinical Professor of Medicine
New York Medical College
New York, New York
President, American College of
  Gastroenterology

Arthur E. Lindner, MD
Associate Professor of Medicine
New York University School of
  Medicine
New York, New York

Jerry Nagler, MD
Assistant Adjunct Physician
  (Gastroenterology)
Lenox Hill Hospital
New York, New York

Daniel H. Present, MD
Associate Clinical Professor
Division of Gastroenterology
Mount Sinai School of Medicine of the
City University of New York
New York, New York

Robert R. Rickert, MD
Co-Director
Department of Pathology
Saint Barnabas Medical Center
Livingston, New Jersey, and
Adjunct Associate Professor of
  Pathology
Columbia University College of
  Physicians and Surgeons
New York, New York

Richard D. Robbins, MD
Assistant Adjunct Surgeon
Lenox Hill Hospital
New York, New York

Margaret Roche, RN
Enterostomal Therapist
Lenox Hill Hospital
New York, New York

Heidi Z. Rotterdam, MD
Associate Pathologist
Lenox Hill Hospital
New York, New York

Irving A. Rubin
President
National Foundation for Ileitis and
  Colitis, Inc.
Detroit, Michigan

David B. Sachar, MD
Associate Professor of Medicine
Mount Sinai School of Medicine of the
City University of New York
New York, New York

Michael J. Schmerin, MD
Assistant Adjunct Physician
  (Gastroenterology)
Lenox Hill Hospital
New York, New York

Norman Sohn, MD
Adjunct Surgeon
Lenox Hill Hospital
New York, New York

Sheldon C. Sommers, MD
Director of Laboratories
Lenox Hill Hospital, and
Clinical Professor of Pathology
Columbia University College of
  Physicians and Surgeons
New York, New York

Felicien M. Steichen, MD
Director of Surgery
Lenox Hill Hospital
Professor of Surgery
New York Medical College
New York, New York

Jerome D. Waye, MD
Attending Physician (Gastroenterology)
Lenox Hill Hospital, and
Associate Clinical Professor
Department of Medicine
Mount Sinai School of Medicine of the
City University of New York, and
Chief, Gastrointestinal Endoscopy Unit
Mount Sinai Hospital
New York, New York

Michael A. Weinstein, MD
Adjunct Surgeon
Lenox Hill Hospital
New York, New York

Nathaniel Wisch, MD
Chief of Hematology
Lenox Hill Hospital, and
Associate Clinical Professor
Department of Medicine
Mount Sinai School of Medicine of the
City University of New York
New York, New York

CONTENTS

SPECIAL PRESENTATION

Medicine is an ever-changing science. As new research and clinical experience broaden our knowledge, changes in treatment and drug therapy are required. The author and the publisher of this work have made every effort to ensure that the treatment and drug dosage schedules herein is accurate and in accord with the standards accepted at the time of publication. Readers are advised, however, to check the product information sheet included in the package of each drug they plan to administer to be certain that changes have not been made in the recommended dose or in the indications and contraindications for administration. This recommendation is of particular importance in regard to new or infrequently used drugs.

INTRODUCTION

Grouping ulcerative colitis with Crohn's disease (Inflammatory Bowel Disease) in a teaching seminar has historical support. The medical literature includes descriptions of both diseases in the latter half of the 19th century; they share many symptoms; in some instances, differentiating them may be very difficult; and the cause of each remains unknown. Furthermore, one member of a family may suffer with Crohn's disease while another has ulcerative colitis. And both processes are prone to the late complications of carcinoma at a site of previous involvement. Finally, the investigators and students of one disease have usually also contributed to the understanding of the other disease.

The incidence of Crohn's disease seems to be increasing rapidly. This has been suggested by reports from Sweden, the Netherlands, England, Scotland, and South Africa as well as the United States. Though methods of recording data vary, the increase is further supported by cases of greater virulence, still younger ages of onset, and more cases in the elderly. This is remarkable when we consider that fifty years ago, when the classic description from Mt. Sinai Hospital was being prepared, the disease was rare. Since the cause remains elusive, we must try to cope with this entity as skillfully as we can, with consideration of indications, and timing of drug and surgical intervention. The choice of forms of management has been controversial, even among the most experienced physicians.

The incidence of ulcerative colitis seems to be stable. Nonsurgical management has improved, however, so that surgery under urgent circumstances is not required as often. Many patients now have the opportunity to have a continent ileostomy when surgery can be performed electively. However, successful nonsurgical management has also created a greater likelihood of developing carcinoma of the rectum or colon. These considerations also introduce controversy.

The accumulated experience of the participants in this seminar is vast. It represents a background of concerted interest and study in inflammatory bowel disease at the Cleveland Clinic, The Johns Hopkins Hospital, Mount Sinai Hospital, New York University School of Medicine, St. Barnabas Medical Center, the National Foundation for Ileitis and Colitis, and Lenox Hill Hospital. Many disciplines and physicians of varied specialties are represented in these proceedings. Lenox Hill is proud to present this course on inflammatory bowel disease.

Burton I. Korelitz, MD

1 The History of Crohn's Disease

Harry D. Fein, MD

It is probable that Morgagni, as early as 1769 in *De Sedibus et Causis Morborum,* ("The Seats and Causes of Diseases"), gave the first clinical description of a case of Crohn's disease. In 1865, probably the first clinical and pathological description of ulcerative colitis was recorded in the annals of the Union Army Medical Corps. It was not until 1909 that Braun described several cases of inflammatory disease masses involving the small intestine. Dalziel in 1913 reported, in detail, six cases similar to those of Braun, in which tuberculosis (though suspected) was excluded by careful bacteriological studies. This evoked some acceptance that a benign, chronic, granulomatous condition of the small intestine existed which was not tuberculosis.

However, for most of us, the history of this disease really started in 1932. On May 13, 1932, in New Orleans, a paper by Crohn, Ginzburg and Oppenheimer was read before the Section of Gastroenterology and Proctology at the 83rd Session of the American Medical Association. It was entitled "Regional Enteritis, a Pathological and Clinical Entity." The authors proposed to describe in its pathological and clinical details, "a disease of the terminal ileum affecting mainly young adults, characterized by a

1

subacute or chronic, necrotizing and cicatrizing inflammation." They stated that "the ulceration of the mucosa is accompanied by a disproportionate connective tissue reaction of the remaining walls of the involved intestine, a process which frequently leads to stenosis of the lumen of the intestine and is associated with multiple fistulas." To further quote, "The disease is clinically featured by symptoms that resemble those of ulcerative colitis; namely, fever, diarrhea, and emaciation leading eventually to an obstruction of the small intestine. The constant occurrence of a mass in the right iliac fossa usually requires surgical intervention, that is, resection. The terminal ileum alone is involved." The process begins abruptly at and involves the ileocecal valve in its maximum intensity, tapering off gradually as it ascends the ileum proximally for 20 to 30 cm. The familiar fistulas usually lead to segments of the colon forming small tracts communicating with the lumen of the large intestine. Occasionally the anterior abdominal wall is the site of one or more of these fistulous tracts. Continuing quotes of that paper, "The etiology of the process is unknown" and perhaps we have not advanced too far in that direction. "It belongs in none of the categories of recognized granulomatous or accepted inflammatory groups, the course is relatively benign, all the patients who survive operations being alive and well." Such, in essence, is the definition of a disease. The description is based on a study of 14 cases up to 1932.

We then made some progress when in 1949 Dr Crohn, in a monograph, indicated that regional ileitis was a better term than terminal ileitis, as the first 14 cases were named. It denotes a much more widespread distribution. Ileocolitis was introduced to denote the frequent involvement of the colon. Then ileojejunitis came about to include anatomically all the jejunum continuously or sequentially, and finally coloileitis.

It should be mentioned, however, that as early as 1923, and again in 1927 Drs Moschowitz and Wilensky described four cases of benign intestinal granuloma, detailing one case involving the terminal ileum which closely resembled that in Crohn's original description.

More recently, a monograph entitled "Crohn's Disease," by Brook, Cave, Gurry and King, published in 1977, indicated that in a review of the history of the subject, 16 different eponymous terms had been listed, reflecting the protean manifestations and interpretations of the disease.

In the absence of any known etiology, definition is of necessity based on a synthesis of clinical, radiological, and pathological criteria. Such a definition provides a framework for discussion and distinguishes Crohn's disease from ulcerative colitis. There is some overlap, although their interrelationship remains obscure. Crohn's disease is a chronic, progressive, granulomatous disorder which can affect the gastrointestinal tract from mouth to anus. Secondary lesions may involve regional lymph nodes, liver, skin, eyes and joints. The cellular reaction in the intestine is transmural and consists of hyperplasia of histiocytic cells associated with acute and chronic inflammatory cells and lymphoid aggregates. The histiocytes may coalesce to form Langhans type giant cells and noncaseating granulomas. Ulceration of the mucosa and deep fissures which lead to fistula formation are present. Microscopically, its anatomical discontinuity, skip lesions, a tendency to fistula formation, and a very high incidence of recurrence after surgery are the hallmarks of the disease. The radiologic changes reflect the macroscopic changes, and although they are of some value diagnostically, they may not be of definitive help.

Since the theme of this symposium is experience and controversy, I would like to introduce a little element of controversy, even in the historical background. Actually, Dr Crohn had observed only two cases of the original 14 cases reported. Most of the cases had been carefully studied by Dr Ginzburg, whose interest was aroused in this subject as early as 1925. He was a house surgeon, then an adjunct, and then Dr A. A. Berg's assistant in private practice. Those who knew Dr Berg as the Chief of Surgery, or knew of him, knew that aside from his tremendous skill as a surgeon with an enormous private practice, he was also quite an autocrat. It was his idea that Dr Crohn's name be listed among the authors of the paper. It was also his feeling that the names should be in alphabetical order. Thus, Crohn came first, and Crohn's disease was born. Dr Berg declined to have his own name on the paper, or we might be talking about Berg's disease. However, it became Crohn's disease.

BIBLIOGRAPHY

Braun H: Veber entzunollische Geschwultse, am Darm. *Dtsch Z Chin* 100:1, 1909.

Brooke BN, Cave DR, Gurry JF, et al: *Crohn's Disease*. New York, Oxford University Press, 1977.

Crohn B, Ginzburg L, Oppenheimer GD: Regional ileitis. *JAMA* 99:1323, 1932.

Dalziel TK: Chronic interstitial enteritis. *Br Med J* 2:1068, 1913.

Morgagni GB: *De Sedibus et Causis Morborum (The Seats and Causes of Disease)*. London, Millar and Cadwell, 1769. Facsimile of the 1769 edition. New York, Hafner, 1960.

Moschowitz E, Wilensky A: Nonspecific granulomata of the intestine. *Am J Med Sci* 166:48, 1923.

Moschowitz E, Wilensky A: Nonspecific granulomata of the intestine. *Am J Med Sci* 178:374, 1927.

Union Army Medical Corps: *Medical and Surgical History of the Rebellion, USA:* Washington, Circular No. 6, 1865, p 139.

2 An Internist's View of Inflammatory Bowel Disease

Michael S. Bruno, MD

My premise has always been that an internist should have a broad view of the spectrum of diseases which he sees, and a comprehensive knowledge of the more common conditions. Inflammatory bowel disease is an important disease in medicine, with an incidence that appears to be increasing tremendously. This has been our experience at Lenox Hill Hospital, no doubt because we have so many physicians who are interested in the problem. The most crucial role for the internist when faced with the problem of inflammatory bowel disease is proper identification. Since patients often see internists as their primary physician, it is the internist who has the responsibility of first making the correct diagnosis. It is hoped that he will make that diagnosis as early as possible, in spite of the protean nature of these diseases and the way they can present at any given point in time. Among the conditions that often have to be considered in the group classified as the chronic diarrheas, ulcerative colitis and Crohn's disease are two of the most important. In addition, we often have to consider enterocolitis of specific infectious etiology, including amebiasis, which we see frequently. If overlooked or confused with one or the other of the two conditions we are discussing, and left untreated, amebiasis may be potentially catastrophic.

The bacillary dysenteries and giardiasis are also being seen with increasing frequency, particularly in New York City. Also to be considered in the differential diagnosis of the chronic diarrheal states is ischemic colitis, with its characteristic radiographic features seen in certain elderly groups. Its clinical picture is similar to that of certain types of Crohn's disease and perhaps even ulcerative colitis. Lastly, we must consider enterocolitis associated with administering some of our newer antibiotics, especially lincomycin and clindamycin.

As an introduction to the problems of ulcerative colitis and Crohn's disease, I shall briefly present a clinical overview of both these conditions, considering the basic pathology and pathophysiology, while emphasizing the variability of these diseases and their more important intestinal and the extraintestinal manifestations. As I see it, the role of the internist should be to identify these diseases when first seen, to sequester them from the other conditions mentioned, and to treat the majority of them appropriately if it is within his ability to do so. The extent of his role in the management of cases of inflammatory bowel disease comes down to interest and to experience.

Ulcerative colitis is a confluent, erosive, inflammatory process which is symmetrical and specifically involves the mucosal surfaces of the colon. It may occasionally extend beyond the mucosa to involve the submucosa, but it is basically a mucosal disease. It most commonly involves the rectum, rectosigmoid and left colon. In many of the cases, the distribution of the disease process stops abruptly at the mid-transverse colon for reasons that are not apparent. Approximately 30% of these patients have total involvement of the colon; half of this group also have involvement of the terminal ileum. When that is the case, radiographic differentiation from Crohn's disease may be difficult. The most common distribution of ulcerative colitis, of course, is ulcerative proctitis. Some physicians separate these two conditions, but most feel that they are the same disease process. While ulcerative proctitis can be very invasive and destructive, for reasons that we do not entirely understand, the condition usually remains localized, rarely extending beyond this segment of the bowel. While the process is quite invasive and destructive locally, these patients can do quite well, can continue to work and be fully productive, being seen as office patients almost exclusively. Patients with this disease are rarely brought into the hospital except perhaps to establish the diagnosis. The true incidence, therefore, is not too well known. While local therapy often suffices, these cases can be very resistant to therapy.

I am not going to discuss the etiology of ulcerative colitis in any detail; it will be discussed by others. Certainly ethnic, emotional, environmental, and autoimmune factors are to be considered. We still do not know the cause of ulcerative colitis. Some of these patients have elevated circulating immunoglobulins, others may have high antibody titers against colonic epithelium. What role autoimmunity, environment, stress and ethnic background play in the etiology of these diseases will be discussed further by others.

Pathologically, ulcerative colitis is also a mucosal process. The mucosa is confluently ulcerated with residual mucosal bridges; sometimes there is complete effacement of the mucosa. Pseudopolyps are an important pathologic feature of this disease, due to hypertrophy of some of the residual islets of colonic mucosa. While the submucosa is involved in some instances, ulcerative colitis is basically a symmetrical confluent mucosal disease. Crypt abscesses are prominent and the exudative process is primarily due to a leukocytic infiltration; there is a decrease in the mucous goblet cells and an increase in the numbers of mass cells. Rectal biopsy is extremely important in differentiating ulcerative colitis from Crohn's disease, but may not always be definitive. These patients usually have a history of bloody diarrhea. The physical examination can vary from the mild case where there are no physical findings, to the severe forms of the disease, where the patient may be overwhelmed with prominent intestinal and extraintestinal manifestations. The internist continually has to be aware of the widespread nature of this disease process and the variable presenting complaints and physical findings. Sigmoidoscopy and biopsy are extremely important; barium enema has obvious indications. Stool cultures should be done in every case and stools should be repeatedly examined for ova and parasites. Identifying the occasional case of amebiasis or other parasitic infestation which can mimic this disease can spare lives. Complement fixation and hemagglutination tests for amebiasis should always be done. I won't dwell on the local complications of ulcerative colitis, but I would like to comment on some of the systemic manifestations. These are often the complaints that bring the patient to the internist, to the ophthalmologist, or to the rheumatologist. These patients may have a polyarthritis or polyarthralgia that is prominent, severe and debilitating, suggesting the diagnosis of rheumatoid arthritis. The intestinal symptoms at any one time may be subtle, if at all present, and an incorrect diagnosis of a rheumatoid-like state can be made. These patients often have a prominent erythema nodosum. Uveitis is a very important feature of this disease and may precede the development of all intestinal complaints, first bringing the patient to the ophthalmologist. Since uveitis can persist even after total colectomy and the successful removal of the disease process, one has to wonder about the persistence of circulating antibodies. Pyoderma gangrenosa, nephrolithiasis, and pericholangitis are other features of this disease when seen in its more severe form.

The systemic manifestations of ulcerative colitis usually parallel the severity of the disease, may precede bowel symptoms by years (uveitis), and may persist after successful total colectomy (uveitis and pericholangitis).

Granulomatous colitis, or Crohn's disease, was originally described as an inflammatory process involving only the terminal ileum. It is now recognized as a disease which involves any segment of the gastrointestinal tract from the mouth to the anus, with or without involvement of the terminal ileum. Ileocolitis is the most common form of the disease, and it is much more common than disease restricted to the terminal ileum.

It is important to emphasize that anal symptoms are often the presenting problem, and that the true incidence of anorectal Crohn's disease is something that has only recently been documented.

Pathologically, Crohn's disease is an inflammatory process which involves the submucosa rather than the mucosa. Granuloma or microgranuloma are found in approximately 50% of all cases. Transverse fissuring and lymphoid hyperplasia and lymphangiectasia, and crypt abscesses containing eosinophils and macrophages are not uncommon. Fistulous tract formation is not only common, but is one of the most devastating features of this process. Skip areas of involvement are very common, as well as stricture formation and obstruction. There are many clinical similarities between Crohn's disease and ulcerative colitis, including the development of massive gastrointestinal hemorrhage and toxic megacolon.

The disease process may be very protean in its presentation. Afflicted patients often present with developmental defects, symptoms of malabsorption syndrome, and nutritional deficiencies. Anorexia, weight loss, and fever of unknown origin are often presenting complaints in these patients. Patients usually have persistent, nonbloody diarrhea, abdominal cramps, low grade fever, anorexia, malaise, or a combination of these. Patients afflicted with Crohn's disease may also have erythema nodosum, iritis, polyarthritis, pyoderma gangrenosum, fistulae, and intraabdominal abscess, especially pelvic abscess associated with the fistulae and small bowel obstruction. When present, these usually represent rather advanced disease.

On physical examination, these patients may look cachectic and malnourished and present a picture of chronic or severe illness. An abdominal mass is not uncommon, and when present is usually in the lower quadrants or in the pelvis. The sigmoidoscopic findings will be presented later.

Rectal biopsy is extremely important and is required in all cases. Although the rectal mucosa may appear normal on gross inspection, careful pathological study of the biopsy material may reveal significant changes. Even with what appears to be normal rectal mucosa, significant abnormalities are found in at least 30% of cases with a number showing granuloma or microgranuloma. Rectal mucosal biopsy is therefore extremely important in establishing the diagnosis, in differentiating this condition from others with a rectal component, and certainly in monitoring the activity of the disease. Barium study of the entire gastrointestinal tract is also very important diagnostically for any patient suspected of having Crohn's disease.

The internist or primary physician should be aware of the natural history of these diseases. In the management of inflammatory bowel disease, he will either be the first or one of the first physicians to see these patients. He ought to be fully aware of the diagnostic possibilities and the variability of the presenting complaints, including the extraintestinal manifestations of the disease, which may be the presenting or dominant complaint. He must anticipate some of the complications of these diseases, ie, carcinoma in ulcerative colitis, fistulous tracts, and intraabdominal abscesses in moderately severe or severe forms of Crohn's disease. He must be able to manage these conditions intelligently and correctly. I believe he ought to be able to care for the majority of these patients properly. When the circumstances dictate, he must be able to identify the potentially lethal complications quickly, and, when present, refer them to individuals who by training and experience can handle them most appropriately.

3 Evidence for Crohn's Disease As an Extensive Process

Burton I. Korelitz, MD

Crohn's disease as originally described was called terminal ileitis and its name was later changed to regional ileitis. Soon thereafter it was realized that granulomatous inflammation could involve the other side of the ileocecal valve, the colon. In fact, it could involve the entire colon, and this distribution was initially referred to in New York as granulomatous colitis. Soon after there was increasing emphasis on Crohn's disease involving the anal structures. There are characteristic anal skin tabs, referred to by Dr Sohn, our colon and rectal surgeon, as "elephant ears." When we see these, we know that they are diagnostic of Crohn's disease. We know now that Crohn's disease can involve the ileum, the colon, and the anal structures. We know it can manifest itself in the form of diffuse jejunoileitis. Furthermore, we have learned that it can involve the stomach alone, the stomach with the duodenum, or the duodenum alone. We know that the esophagus infrequently can be involved with Crohn's disease. Furthermore, characteristic lesions have been found along the gingivae and on the tongue or lips, with the biopsy showing the characteristic granulomata of Crohn's disease.

Crohn's disease is prone to fistula formation. The fistulae characteristically arise from the zone of maximum involvement and can aim in all directions, the most characteristic arising from the terminal ileum and pointing toward the rectum, toward the sigmoid, into the bladder, the vagina, to other loops of ileum, and into the proximal colon. If the worst area of involvement is a segment of the colon, the fistula can go from this site to other adjoining structures. The most common, independent of the fistulae in and about the anus and rectum, are the ileorectal, ileocecal, and colonic-duodenal fistulae. Figure 3-1 shows one from the distal ascending colon into the elbow of the duodenum.

Crohn's disease manifests itself in other forms such as pyoderma gangrenosum and erythema nodosum. Figure 3-2 is a radiographic sketch that shows many of the features

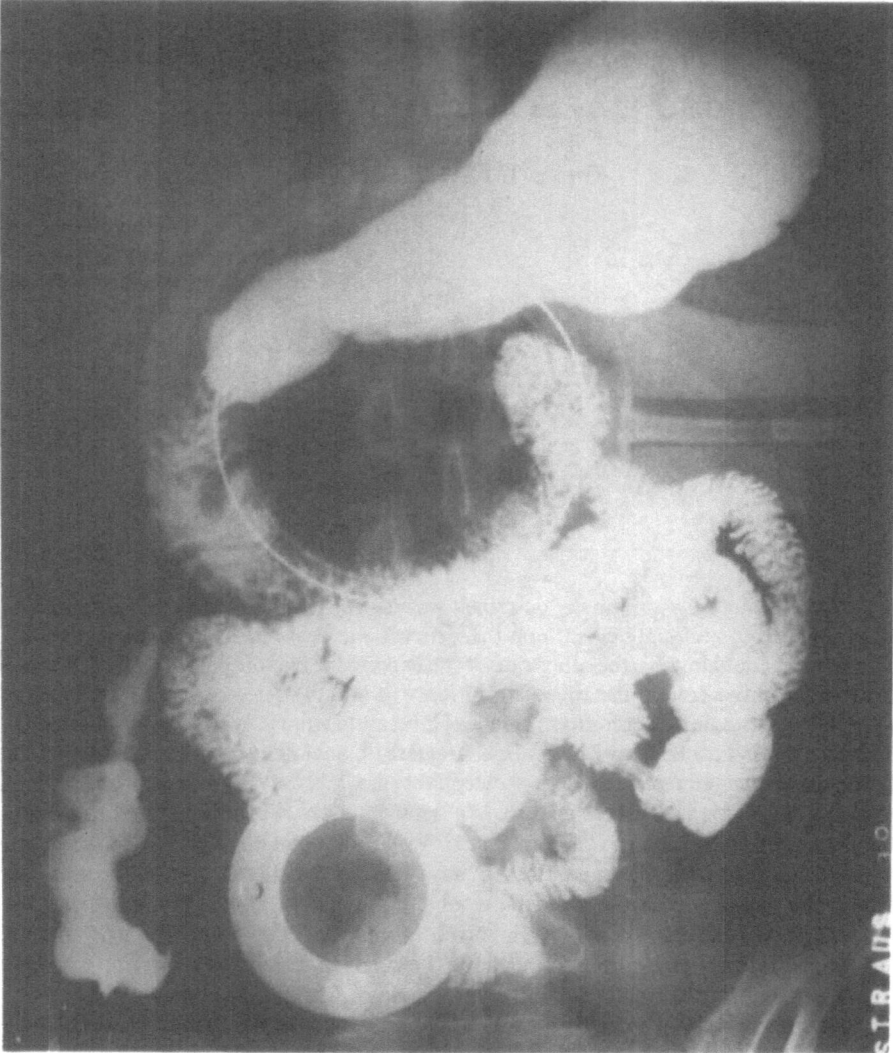

Figure 3-1 Fistula from ascending colon to descending duodenum in Crohn's disease after ileostomy without colectomy.

of Crohn's disease. In its most classic form, the rectal segment is spared. That does not mean that the anus is spared because there can be severe anal disease while the rectal mucosa appears entirely normal. As we proceed proximally (Figure 3-2) one can see an area of fistula formation between the ileum and the rectum. This is a very common one,

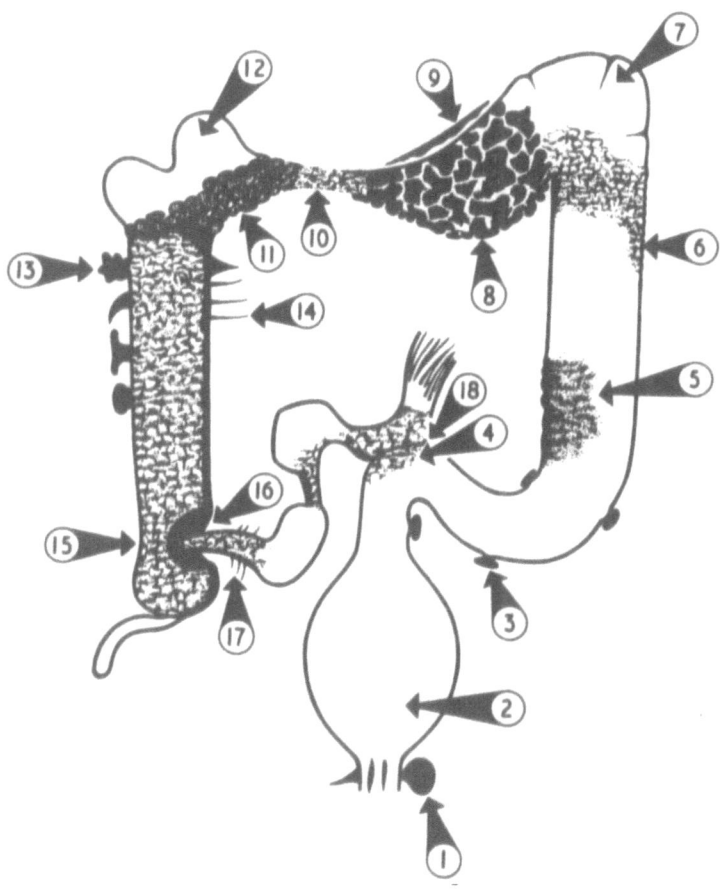

Figure 3-2 The eighteen indicators of Crohn's disease. Features seen on the double-contrast barium enema indicating a diagnosis of Crohn's colitis include: 1) Anal lesions, 2) Normal rectum, 3) Discrete ulcers, 4) Patches of disease surrounded by normal bowel, 5) Aphthous ulceration, 6) Eccentric involvement, 7) Normal patch surrounded by disease, 8) Serpiginous ulceration, 9) Intramural linear ulceration, 10) Stricture, 11) Cobblestone formation, 12) Pouches of normal bowel resulting from contraction of diseased opposite wall, 13) Pleomorphic deep ulceration: composite, horned, collar stud, and saccular, 14) Fissures: raspberry and rose-thorn shaped, deep spicular ulcers, 15) Right-sided disease with contraction of the cecum, 16) Prominent ileocecal value, 17) Small bowel disease, and 18) Fistulae. Courtesy of KC Simpkins, MD, Department of Radiology, Leeds General Infirmary, Leeds, United Kingdom. Reproduced from *Management of Crohn's Disease* (Weterman IT, Pena AS, Booth CC, eds). Amsterdam-Oxford, Excerpta Medica, 1976.

the ileorectal or ileorectosigmoidal fistula. The disease is not confluent as in ulcerative colitis, but rather there may be patches of involvement. There may also be stricture formation, transverse fissures referred to by our British colleagues as "rose thorn lesions." These are the lesions which predispose to fistula formation when there is an adjoining loop of bowel in the proximity. There are also skip areas which appear relatively or completely uninvolved, or the terminal ileum can be involved with rose thorn lesions. The appendix may or may not be part of the process.

The normal-appearing rectal mucosa has been a source of interest to Dr Sommers and me for a long time. In our rectal biopsy study of normal-appearing rectal mucosa in Crohn's disease, we found that 45% of the biopsies showed some abnormality; 30% had lesions which were consistent with the diagnosis of Crohn's disease. In 18% of those normal-appearing rectal mucosal biopsies, we even found granulomas.

In addition to the usual histologic preparations, cell counts of the rectal mucosa were performed. In cases with inflammation that were not Crohn's disease, the cell counts were not very much different from those from noninflammatory cases, and in Crohn's disease there was a significant increase in the number of macrophages. The macrophage count was proportionately more prominent than any other type of histologic feature. This increase in macrophages is another indication that Crohn's disease is an extensive process, despite the fact that the mucosa might appear grossly normal.

We also used this technique at the other end of the alimentary canal. Gastroduodenoscopies were performed on patients with Crohn's disease who had involvement of the ileum and the colon, but in whom the gastrointestinal-series appearance was normal in the upper gastrointestinal tract. Biopsies were taken from the lower esophagus, the body of the stomach, the antrum, and the duodenal bulb. There were gross abnormalities (mostly in the antrum) but, in addition, there were many microscopic abnormalities (also mostly in the antrum). These were relevant in at least half of the cases.

In summary, there were 20% of cases with diagnostic features or features at least consistent with Crohn's disease, whereas others were of possible relevance but not conclusive. Cell counts were also done on these biopsies, and again it was found that the macrophages were increased in Crohn's disease as compared to controls. Mast cells were also increased.

Microscopic lesions were found in the antrum or duodenum in 19 out of 45 cases of Crohn's disease (42%) and about two-thirds of these lesions were thought to be relevant pathologically. Over half were found in normal-appearing mucosa, and all had normal-appearing upper gastrointestinal series. All three granulomas found on these biopsies were located in grossly normal mucosa. There was no correlation with clinical disease activity. Some of these patients were active, some completely inactive.

Other authors have reported results which lead essentially to the same conclusions. Some have found villous abnormalities in the proximal jejunum, lactase-insufficient cells, and increased numbers of plasma cells. A variety of techniques has demonstrated that something is abnormal in the jejunal and ileal mucosa despite the fact that they appear perfectly normal on small bowel x-ray series, and all the demonstrable disease is more distal in the ileum and the colon. We know also that, following any type of surgery for Crohn's disease, there is a recurrence rate of about 15% per year. The explanation for this is not clear, but we have to include in the total concept the possibility that the disease already exists in the normal-appearing tissue and that the surgery merely provokes further activity. All of these findings support the conclusion that Crohn's disease involves the entire alimentary canal from mouth to anus, and it is only at the zones of maximum activity that we are able to visualize the disease with conventional radiography.

BIBLIOGRAPHY

Allan RN, Steinberg DM, Dixon K, et al: Changes in the bidirection sodium flux across the intestinal mucosa in Crohn's disease. *Gut* 16:201–204, 1975.

Carr D: Granulomatous cheilitis in Crohn's disease. *Br Med J* 4:636, 1974.

Chalfin D, Holt PR: Lactase deficiency in ulcerative colitis, regional enteritis and viral hepatitis. *Am J Dig Dis* 12:81–87, 1967.

Comfort MW, Weber HM, Baggenstoss AH, et al: Nonspecific granulomatous inflammation of the stomach and duodenum: its relation to regional enteritis. *Am J Med Sci* 220:616–632, 1950.

Crohn BB, Ginsburg L, Oppenheimer GD: Regional ileitis. *JAMA* 99:1323–1329, 1937.

Dudney TP: Crohn's disease of the mouth. *Proc R Soc Med* 62:1237, 1969.

Dunne WT, Cooke WT, Allan RN: Enzymatic and morphometric evidence for Crohn's disease as a diffuse lesion of the gastrointestinal tract. *Gut* 18:290–294, 1977.

Ferguson R, Allan RN, Cooke WT: The proximal jejunal mucosa in colonic Crohn's disease and ulcerative colitis. *Gut* 16:205–208, 1975.

Fielding JR, Toye DKM, Beton DD, et al: Crohn's disease of the stomach and duodenum. *Gut* 11:1001–1006, 1970.

Gelfand MD, Krone CL: Dysphagia and esophageal ulcerations in Crohn's disease. *Gastroenterology* 55:510–514, 1968.

Glass RE, Baker WNW: Role of the granuloma in recurrent Crohn's disease. *Gut* 17:75–77, 1976.

Goodman MJ, Skiner JM, Truelove SC: Abnormalities in the apparently normal bowel mucosa in Crohn's disease. *Lancet* 1:275–278, 1976.

Gottlieb C, Alpert S: Regional jejunitis. *Am J Roentgenol* 38:771–783, 1937.

Harrer WV, Goldstein F, Wirts CW: Granulomas in suction biopsies of distal duodenum. *Gastroenterology* 59:862–867, 1970.

Hermos JA, Cooper HL, Kramer P, et al: Histological diagnosis peroral biopsy of Crohn's disease of the proximal intestines. *Gastroenterology* 59:868–873, 1970.

Korelitz BI: Clinical course, late results, and pathological nature of the inflammatory disease of the colon initially sparing the rectum. *Gut* 8:281–290, 1967.

Korelitz BI, Sommers SC: Differential diagnosis of ulcerative and granulamatous colitis by sigmoidoscopy, rectal biopsy and cell counts of rectal mucosa. *Am J Gastroenterol* 61:460–469, 1974.

Korelitz BI, Present DH, Alpert LK, et al: Recurrent regional ileitis after ileostomy and colectomy for granulomatous colitis. *N Engl J Med* 287:110–115, 1972.

Korelitz BI, Sommers SC: Rectal biopsy in patients with Crohn's disease. Normal mucosa on sigmoidoscopic examination. *JAMA* 237:2742–2744, 1977.

Korelitz BI, Waye JD, Kreuning J, et al: Crohn's disease in endoscopy biopsies of the gastric antrum and duodenum. Submitted for publication.

Madden JL, Ravid JM, Haddad JR: Regional esophagitis: a specific entity simulating Crohn's disease. *Ann Surg* 170:351–368, 1969.

14

Nugent FW, Richmond M, Park SK: Crohn's disease of the duodenum. *Gut* 18:115–120, 1977.

Richman A, Zeifer HD, Winkelstein A, et al: Chronic non-specific granulomatous inflammation of the stomach, duodenum and intestine. *Gastroenterology* 29:358–369, 1955.

Rotterdam H, Korelitz BI, Sommers SC: Microgranulomas in grossly normal rectal mucosa in Crohn's disease. *Am J Clin Path* 67:550–554, 1977.

Shiner M, Drury RA: Abnormalities of the small intestine mucosa in Crohn's disease (regional enteritis). *Am J Dig Dis* 7:744–759, 1962.

Sommers SC, Korelitz BI: Mucosal cell counts in ulcerative and granulomatous colitis. *Am J Clin Path* 63:349–365, 1975.

4 Implications of Uveitis and Other Extraintestinal Manifestations of Inflammatory Bowel Disease

Robert S. Coles, MD

Reviewing a group of patients with inflammatory bowel disease (IBD) in a paper we published several years ago,[1] we found that there was a wide spectrum of ocular complications associated with inflammatory bowel disease, ranging from episcleritis to conjunctivitis, orbital cellulitis, proptosis, and uveitis. But of all the many ophthalmic complications associated with inflammatory bowel disease, the most interesting and common one was uveitis.

Uveitis is an inflammation which involves the middle layer of the eye, the choroid posteriorly, and the ciliary body and the iris anteriorly. Inflammations of the eye can be divided into anterior uveitis involving the iris (iritis) and the ciliary body (iridocyclitis), and posterior uveitis involving the choroid (choroiditis). Most inflammations involving the anterior portions of the eye are probably immunologic in nature and represent some disturbance in the internal homeostatic mechanism, whereas involvement of the posterior portion is probably secondary to invasion by microorganisms. Therefore, the relationship between iritis and inflammatory bowel disease probably is on the same basis as an immunologic disturbance.

The patient who presents with conjunctivitis must be questioned very carefully to determine whether or not the disease is not, in reality, an iridocyclitis or iritis. Such a patient will exhibit marked blepharospasm, have pain radiating around the eye similar to headache, and will complain of lacrimation. The eyes will be extremely red, much more so than in a case of conjunctivitis. If one examines a patient with acute iritis with a sudden, painful onset, there is marked injection of the limbus, diminishing toward the cul-de-sac. With a slitlamp, one can see keratic precipitates (KP's) on the cornea, which are deposits of inflammatory cells on the endothelium. There may also be a flare and cells in the anterior chamber, similar to Tyndall's phenomenon in which a light beam coming through a dark room is seen as a ray of light against a dark background. The iris itself is edematous and miotic; nodules may be present, and subjectively the patient will be most uncomfortable.

In our study there were several interesting correlations. Of the 13 patients with iridocyclitis and inflammatory bowel disease, the most important observation was that most of the patients managed to maintain fairly good vision throughout the entire course of the disease, except for two, one who became totally blind, and the other whose vision was reduced to hand motions. Another conclusion of that study was that no temporal correlation existed between the appearance of the inflammatory reaction involving the eye and the inflammatory reaction involving the gut. In many instances the two diseases appeared simultaneously, and at other times they presented asynchronously without any particular correlation. Indeed, in those patients who lost their vision, the cases with the worst prognosis, the colitis was quiescent while the ocular inflammation persisted in a chronic form. On the other hand, some patients had recurrent episodes of uveitis with no loss of vision, both with and without active colitis, indicating a lack of any causal relationship between inflammatory activity in the bowel and inflammatory activity in the eye. The two organs appear to act asynchronously and independently when they are involved.

Table 4-1 shows that in four instances the uveitis preceded the occurrence of the inflammatory bowel disease by many years. This is particularly significant in terms of management. It has been suggested that if inflammatory bowel disease is present, it is important to eradicate this focus of infection and thus cure the iritis. This always has appeared to me as being illogical since, once the disease has become manifest, removal of the other presumed exciting organ is not going to eliminate it because the reaction is an immunologic one. Following this reasoning ad absurdum, it can be stated that, if removal of the bowel will cure the eye disease, why not take the four patients whose eye disease presented prior to their IBD and remove their eye, thus preventing the bowel inflammation from occurring! Such reasoning is analogous and equally specious. In our limited experience there has been no evidence that removal of the bowel will cure the eye disease or any of the other extraintestinal manifestations.

The second interesting observation made in our study was that, while we did not know of the existence of the histocompatibility antigens at that time, we found that there was one group of patients who presented with a triad of arthritis, inflammatory bowel disease, and iritis; and another group who had a triad of erythema nodosum or other skin manifestation, inflammatory bowel disease, and iritis. These were two distinct patient populations. Those patients who had one extraintestinal manifestation were at much greater risk to develop a second extraintestinal manifestation. In other words, one could separate the group of patients who had iritis, skin disease, and joint manifestations from those who had inflammatory bowel disease without these extraintestinal manifestations. The incidence of erythema nodosum is about 5%. In our group of patients with uveitis, it was 30%. The expected incidence of arthritis complicating IBD is about 36%; in our group it approached 90%. Thus these were significantly different groups of patients in terms of their reaction to the inflammatory bowel disease. Patients with IBD who presented with one extraintestinal manifestation were at much greater risk of developing other extrabowel manifestations simultaneously. There is some common immunologic predilection for these patients to have multisystem involvement concomitant with IBD. This could be a genetic predisposition, as may eventually be demonstrated by histocompatibility studies.

Recently, Greenstein and associates[2] reviewed 700 patients who had inflammatory bowel disease and listed the changes that occurred in the skin, the joints, and the eye, in terms of frequency of manifestation. They were able to divide their patients into three

Table 4-1
Iritis and Ulcerative Colitis

NAME	AGE ONSET: COLITIS	UVEITIS	RELATIONSHIP ONSET COLITIS TO IRITIS	OTHER SYSTEMIC COMPLICATIONS
E. W. 133178	15 yrs.	17 yrs.	+ 2 yrs.	ARTHRALGIAS ERYTHEMA NODOSUM
P. G. 24419	1 1/2 yrs.	11 yrs.	+ 9 yrs.	NONE
T. B. 64747	38 yrs.	36 yrs.	− 2 yrs.	ARTHRALGIAS ERYTHEMA NODOSUM
N. T. 28345	18 yrs.	17 yrs.	− 1 yr.	POLYARTHRITIS APHTHOUS STOMATITIS
S. W. 56101	22 yrs.	27 yrs.	+ 5 yrs.	ARTHRITIS
D. G. 2672	40 yrs.	44 yrs.	+ 4 yrs.	ARTHRITIS ERYTHEMA NODOSUM
S. F. 52965	35 yrs.	40 yrs.	+ 5 yrs.	ARTHRITIS
L. D.	26 yrs.	20 yrs.	− 6 yrs.	ARTHRITIS ERYTHEMA NODOSUM
C. W.	37 yrs.	44 yrs.	+ 7 yrs.	ARTHRITIS
A. T.	30 yrs.	35 yrs.	+ 5 yrs.	ARTHRITIS
B. S.	25 yrs.	43 yrs.	+ 18 yrs.	ARTHRITIS
M. F. 518056	29 yrs.	9 yrs.	− 20 yrs.	ARTHRITIS

groups. Those in Group A were colitis-related, Group B was related to pathophysiology of the small bowel, and a nonspecific Group C which was very small. Most of our patients were in Group A. These are the patients who have most of the extraintestinal manifestations.

Greenstein and his colleagues[2] found the highest incidence of complications in patients whose colon was involved. Joint manifestations were present in 39% of patients with Crohn's disease and 26% in the ulcerative colitis group. Skin manifestations ranged from 19% to 23%, and eye lesions from 4% to 13%. The predominant skin lesion was erythema nodosum, and was more frequent in the patients with colonic involvement: an incidence of 15% in the granulomatous and 4% in the ulcerative colitis group. The second most common finding was pyoderma gangrenosum, which was higher in the ulcerative colitis group as opposed to the Crohn's disease group, a reversal of our previous findings.

The arthritic manifestations are of two varieties. First, there is polyarthritis, which is monarticular and usually involves the lower limbs. This is much more common in patients with granulomatous colitis as opposed to those with ulcerative colitis, but it does occur in both groups. Spondylitis is the second most important finding. Those patients with HLA antigens are the ones at greatest risk of developing this complication.[3]

Table 4-3[3] indicates that patients with inflammatory bowel disease are at greater risk of developing extraintestinal manifestations of their disease if they have a positive HLA B27. Fifty-six percent of patients with inflammatory bowel disease and arthritis have positive HLA B27 antigens, and in those with juvenile onset arthritis, the figure is 42%. This group also has a high incidence of iritis. These two groups of patients have a high association with uveitis; the common factor between them is the presence of the HLA B27 antigen.

Table 4-3 demonstrates that the incidence of ankylosing spondylitis in B27-positive individuals in the general population is about 3% and that patients with Crohn's disease

Table 4-2
Summary of the Frequency of W27 Antigen in Published Reports of Different Forms of Arthritis

	No. of Patients	% Positive Range	Grand Mean, %	Positive for W27 Antigen and Sacroiliitis,* %	Positive for W27 Antigen and only Peripheral Arthritis,* %
Ankylosing spondylitis	220	81-100	92	...	...
Reiter syndrome	162	57-96	80	100 (6/6)	...
Inflammatory bowel disease arthritis	49	50-75	56	67 (23/41)	6 (1/16)
Juvenile onset arthritis	26	42	42	...	...
Psoriasis and arthritis	118	7-63	31	50 (13/26)	17 (10/59)
Controls	...	4-13	...	...	...

*When specified.

Modified with permission from Mills DM, Yosh A, and Ramesh: *JAMA* 231:268–270, 1975.

without B27 have a still lower incidence. The ulcerative colitis group has an incidence of only 5%. However, if the patients with ulcerative colitis also have B27, the incidence increases to 40%. These patients are also at much greater risk to develop iritis and skin lesions.[4]

It would seem that the group of patients who have certain antigenic moieties as determined genetically by the HLA factor are at much greater risk to develop extraintestial manifestations. Perhaps, eventually, we can subdivide inflammatory bowel diseases on a genetic basis by their predilection for certain types of inflammation involving the bowel and extraintestinal sites, using HLA loci. There may be an infectious agent similar to the HLA that might exert its influence through this route because of nonrecognition on the part of the host.

Table 4-3
Relative Risk of Developing Ankylosing Spondylitis (%)

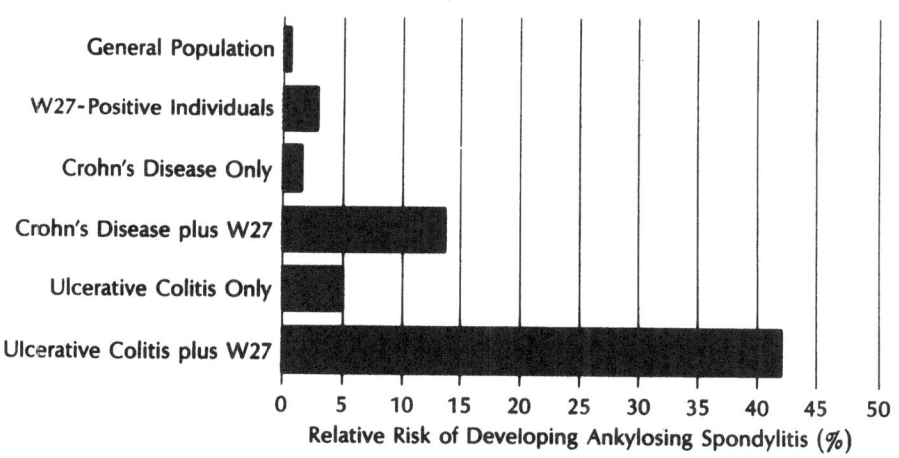

Relative Risk of Developing Ankylosing Spondylitis (%)

Reproduced with permission from *Hospital Practice,* April 1975, p 135.

REFERENCES

1. Korelitz BI, Coles RS: Uveitis (iritis) with ulcerative and granulomatous colitis. *Gastroenterology* 52:78, 1967.

2. Greenstein AJ, Janowitz HD, Sachar ED: The extraintestinal complications of Crohn's disease and ulcerative colitis: a study of 700 patients. *Medicine* 55:401, 1976.

3. Mills DM, Yosh A, Ramesh GC: HLA antigens and sacroiliitis. *JAMA* 231:268–270, 1975.

4. Bluestone R: HL-A W27 and the "rheumatoid variants." *Hosp Practice,* April 1975, p 131.

5 Environment vs Heredity in Inflammatory Bowel Disease

Theodore M. Bayless, MD

In a discussion of the etiology of inflammatory bowel disease (IBD), environment vs heredity can be included. In terms of Crohn's disease, one might consider host characteristics, factors that favor the role of an infectious agent, characteristics of the ideal agent if it were to be found, and the role of an intraluminal agent, ie, the fact that something within the lumen seems to be a major factor. Ulcerative colitis could also be discussed in the same general format of host characteristics, the presumed initial inciting agent or factor that might be involved, the mechanisms that might perpetuate this inflammatory process, perhaps involving prostaglandins, the liability of a fulminative course, perhaps including CMV virus or *Clostridium difficile* toxin in some patients; and the liability to malignant degeneration.

CROHN'S DISEASE

Host Characteristics

What are the host characteristics? These are young people with an average age of 27.

Ten percent had the illness before the age of 15.[1] It is unusual to have the illness present after age 40, and a very small percentage start after age 50. Thus this is an illness that is found in young adults. How young it occurs is not clear. I have a 4-year-old patient, and there have been reports in infants. But I think it is not as common in the very young, under age 4, as ulcerative colitis seems to be.

Genetic Factors

Ten percent of patients have a positive family history, usually a first-degree relative. Some of the relatives have ulcerative colitis. There have been some family studies by competent observers who feel that one family member has ulcerative colitis and another has Crohn's disease. There is clearly a strong family history in some patients. An interesting factor is that at times one sees the same distribution of disease. I take care of two sisters, both of whom have a very localized patch of Crohn's disease in the rectosigmoid about 4 inches long with an identical appearance. Another example is a father and son who had the same three skip areas in the colon so that you could superimpose their x-ray films. This is a diffuse disease, but why should it manifest so similarly in some families? Population differences have been reported with an incidence of 8 to 10 per 100,000. It is more common in Jewish populations and less so in blacks. In Israel, Crohn's disease is more common in the European or Ashkenazi Jews, and less in the Sephardic or Oriental Jews. It is not clear whether Crohn's disease is rare in Asia.

Psychological Factors

I do not believe that such factors are primary. I think that stress obviously has been involved in some flare-ups in some patients but there does not seem to be any primary personality disorder.

Possible Infectious Etiology

The factors favoring the role for an infectious agent include the increasing prevalence throughout the Western world. While the prevalence of ulcerative colitis is remaining unchanged, Crohn's disease is definitely increasing. This is not just due to better diagnosis; it is a real phenomenon.

The next point is the focal microscopic lesions which have already been discussed. Are these early lesions of Crohn's disease? Perhaps this is where a microorganism is getting started. I think of this as a mucosal lesion, starting in the mucosa and then spreading deeper into the submucosa.

Aphthoid lesions which occur over lymphoid tissue have been described. Is the specialized epithelium above the lymphoid tissue more susceptible to the absorption of some agent? Typhoid fever is perhaps an analogy, where the organism strikes lymphoid tissue. Granulomatous inflammation might favor the role of an infectious agent. Serologic studies of families in New Mexico[2] suggest that even family contacts shared antibacterial antibodies, perhaps to a common organism. This is the only current evidence for transmission from patient to patient. Reports of spouses being involved are very rare. There are at least three such reports. With this exception there are very few patient-to-patient transmission reports. Lymphogranuloma venereum-like chlamydial antibodies have also been reported to be increased in people with Crohn's disease.

Improvement following antibiotic therapy suggests some role for microorganisms. Certainly, some people improve with antibiotic therapy.[3,4] We have found them to be helpful in the medical management, and presumably they eliminate some secondary bacterial factor rather than the primary etiologic factors.

Viral isolation studies, initially exciting, are not very encouraging. Control groups also seemed to be involved, and the ability to transfer these agents to animals has not been successful in most laboratories. Also, the animal inoculation studies remain unconvincing in terms of the transmissability of this illness to animals. Although there is a long list of potential infectious agents that have been considered, none has been definitely shown to be involved.

With respect to the characteristics of a proposed agent, it should have a long dormant period because of the late recurrences that occur after surgical resection. The latency period may last years before the recurrence appears after surgery. This tendency to recur may be due to something that is dormant in the mucosa, intermittently inciting inflammation that is suppressible. It heals with dense scarring, leading to an obstructive phase which then becomes an ideal time for surgery. We believe the agent probably enters the mucosa through the lumen. When an ileostomy is performed, colonic disease tends to become less symptomatic. Also, with hyperalimentation and no oral feedings, the intestinal manifestations sometimes tend to improve. Thus one thinks of some intraluminal agent which affects various parts of the gastrointestinal tract.

ULCERATIVE COLITIS

Ulcerative colitis also affects young people but may occur in the elderly more frequently than Crohn's disease. Genetic factors are also involved in at least 10% of patients. Environmental factors seem quite important in the patient with proctitis. One is impressed with the fact that such patients are affected by stress, and relapses seem to be associated with psychological stress. This, in my own experience, is the most clear-cut relationship of psyche to inflammatory bowel disease.

Perhaps ulcerative colitis begins as an insult in the rectal mucosa. We presume this causes a mucositis, and then perpetuating inflammatory processes take over, causing recurrences and remissions. It appears as if there are increased prostaglandins released in the area of the inflammation, perhaps perpetuating the insult. The studies with rectal sulfasalazine and prostaglandin inhibitors may provide some helpful leads. At times, a chronic unremitting pattern can be recognized. Some patients with acute intermittent ulcerative colitis are easy to treat and the illness remits quickly. They are kept on sulfasalazine and the illness stays in remission. Others, despite all therapy, have chronic, unremitting disease activity.

The exacerbating factors which might lead to a fulminant course include aqueous enemas, barium enemas, and antidiarrheal medications. Cytomegalovirus (CMV) has also been incriminated as an aggravating factor in some patients. This virus has been isolated from rectal biopsies in some patients. A rising anti-CMV titer would also be helpful. It has been suggested that CMV may play a role in causing relapses in some patients. This is not thought to be the cause of ulcerative colitis, but acts as an aggravating factor in some. Recently, *Colstridium difficile* toxin has been identified in the stools of some patients in relapse with a subsequent response to vancomycin therapy.[5]

REFERENCES

1. Burbidge EJ, Huang SS, Bayless TM: Clinical manifestations of Crohn's disease in children and adolescents. *Pediatrics* 55:866–871, 1975.

2. Krosmeyer SJ, Williams RCJ, Wilson ID, et al: Lymphocytotoxic antibody in inflammatory bowel disease. *N Engl J Med* 293:1117, 1975.

3. Whitington PF, Barnes HV, Bayless TM: Medical management of Crohn's disease in adolescence. *Gastroenterology* 72:1338–1344, 1977.

4. Moss AA, Carbone JV, Kressel HY: Radiologic and clinical assessment of broad spectrum antibiotic therapy in Crohn's disease. *Am J Radiol* 131:787–794, 1978.

5. LaMont JT, Trnka YM: Therapeutic implications of *Clostridium difficule* toxin during relapse of chronic inflammatory bowel disease. *Lancet* 1:381–383, 1980.

6 Is There an Immunological Contribution to Inflammatory Bowel Disease?

Jerry Nagler, MD

Evidence for the presence of immunological phenomena occurring in inflammatory bowel disease (IBD) is becoming increasingly compelling. A vast array of different approaches have been used to elucidate these phenomena. Unfortunately, however, their significance still remains speculative.

The presence of antibodies directed against human colonic cells in patients with ulcerative colitis was first reported by Broberger and Perlmann at the University of Stockholm in 1959. Comparing ulcerative colitis sera to those of various other illnesses, and using a hemagglutination technique, they showed that the level of antibodies directed against colonic cells is striking in ulcerative colitis. A few years later, similar findings were demonstrated in patients with regional enteritis. However, no significant correlation has been found so far between these antibody titers and the duration or severity of disease, the extent of colonic involvement, or the occurrence of extracolonic manifestations. Furthermore, these antibodies do not seem to be cytotoxic even in the presence of complement. So, although these antibodies are present, what role they play in the disease process is unknown.

Recently, cytotoxic antibodies directed against lymphocytes in the sera of both ulcerative colitis and regional enteritis patients have been detected by Korsmeyer and his colleagues at the University of New Mexico. He did familial studies showing this antibody to be slightly more prevalent in first-degree relatives (parents, children, and siblings) than in second-degree relatives. However, comparing household contacts to nonhousehold contacts, there was a significant increase in the level of cytotoxic antibodies. There was a very high titer of cytotoxic antibodies, especially in spouses of inflammatory bowel disease patients. These data have been used to suggest that there might be a common environmental etiologic agent triggering the immunological phenomena.

A different and more controversial approach to the presence of immunological phenomena in inflammatory bowel disease has involved the question of anergy. Sachar and his group at Mount Sinai Hospital demonstrated that lymphocytes from both ulcerative colitis and regional enteritis have a decreased responsiveness to the nonspecific mitogen phytohemagglutinin. This decreased responsiveness, however, again did not correlate with extent, duration, or activity of the disease process. Meuwissen and his associates in Amsterdam confirmed this depressed responsiveness in regional enteritis lymphocytes in vitro and in vivo to a whole host of antigens such as streptokinase-streptodornase, Trichophyton, Candida, mumps, and PPD. This decreased responsiveness of inflammatory bowel disease lymphocytes to nonspecific mitogens may be related to their prior stimulation by normal intestinal antigens and subsequent involvement in the inflammatory process within the gastrointestinal tract. However, Asquith and associates at the University of Chicago found a wide range of responsiveness to phytohemagglutinin in lymphocytes even from normal subjects. They could demonstrate only a trend toward poor lymphocyte response in patients with regional enteritis with moderate to severe activity, but no statistical difference. There was no difference at all in ulcerative colitis patients. Similarly, Bird and Britten in Sweden could find no difference in the responsiveness to phytohemagglutinin or PPD in lymphocytes from regional enteritis patients and normal controls.

Most recent attention in the field of immunology in inflammatory bowel disease has been directed at the role of circulating lymphocytes as the cytotoxic agents. Leukocyte migration inhibition studies have demonstrated the responsiveness of ulcerative colitis lymphocytes to fetal colon and jejunoileal extracts. Regional enteritis lymphocytes do not seem to respond to the colon extract, but migration can be inhibited by purified microsomal and mitochondrial extracts of Crohn's disease colonic cells. Interestingly, both regional enteritis and ulcerative colitis lymphocytes seem to respond to an antigen of the colonic bacterial class Enterobacteriaceae. This has been labeled the Kunin antigen. Hence, it can be inferred that different antigens may be recognized by the lymphocytes of regional enteritis and ulcerative colitis patients, leading to different clinical manifestations. Of further interest is the fact that lymphocytes from normal patients can be induced to become cytotoxic for colonic cells or extracts when incubated with the sera of inflammatory bowel disease patients. In normal subjects, there is little or no evidence of cytotoxicity. However, if lymphocytes of normal subjects are preincubated with the sera of ulcerative colitis or granulomatous colitis patients, there is evidence of increased cytotoxicity, in that 73% of colonic cells survived rather than 93%. But if the sera of ulcerative colitis patients who have already had a colectomy are used, this phenomenon does not seem to occur. It has been inferred that perhaps something in the sera of active inflammatory bowel disease patients is inducing these lymphocytes to act as cytotoxic agents.

The cytotoxicity of mononuclear cells for colonic cells has been elegantly elucidated by Shorter and his group at the Mayo Clinic. They have shown that a class of mononuclear cells, which are neither precisely T or B cell lymphocytes in origin but instead have receptors for the FC fragment of antibodies, appear to be the primary cells involved in these cytotoxic reactions. In measuring the percentage of cytotoxicity in a mixed group of mononuclear cells enriched with T type lymphocytes, the activity is decreased. Similarly, with B-enriched lymphocytes it is also decreased. But with a group of mononuclear cells that have the property of a receptor for the FC fragment of antibody, there is a marked increase. This cell has been labeled the K or "killer" cell. The phenomenon of this type of cytotoxicity is called antibody-induced, cell-mediated cytotoxicity. It appears that antibody-induced, cell-mediated cytotoxicity requires either that the antibody be fixed to the target cell, or that the antibody be present in the serum as antigen-antibody complexes.

The sera of inflammatory bowel disease patients have been shown by several investigators to contain circulating antigen-antibody complexes. This has been demonstrated on the basis of both the ability of complement to precipitate soluble complexes in agar gel and the ability of inflammatory bowel disease sera to inhibit other antigen-antibody induced cytotoxic reactions. What is interesting is that the levels of antigen-antibody complexes in inflammatory bowel disease patients seem to correlate well with disease activity as judged by symptoms, histology, and laboratory tests. Besides inducing lymphocyte cytotoxicity, these complexes may theoretically be responsible for initiating crypt abscesses if they are small, or granulomas and extracolonic manifestations if they are large.

In conclusion, there is a variety of evidence to demonstrate that immunological phenomena occur in patients with inflammatory bowel disease. What remains to be shown is whether these immune phenomena are initiating factors in inflammatory bowel disease, involved in maintaining the pathologic lesions, or simply innocent bystanders.

BIBLIOGRAPHY

Asquith P, Sumner CK, Rothberg RM: Lymphocyte responses to nonspecific mitogens in inflammatory bowel disease. *Gastroenterology* 65:1, 1973.

Bendixen G: Cellular hypersensitivity to components of intestinal mucosa in ulcerative colitis and Crohn's disease. *Gut* 10:631, 1969.

Bird AG, Britton S: No evidence for decreased lymphocyte reactivity in Crohn's disease. *Gastroenterology* 67:926, 1974.

Broberger O, Perlmann P: Autoantibodies in human ulcerative colitis. *J Exp Med* 110:657, 1959.

Deodhar SD, Michener WM, Farmer RG: A study of the immunologic aspects of chronic ulcerative colitis and transmural colitis. *Am J Clin Path* 51:591, 1969.

Doe WF, Booth CC, Brown DL: Evidence for complement-binding immune complexes in adult coeliac disease, Crohn's disease, and ulcerative colitis. *Lancet* 1:402, 1973.

Jewell DP, MacLennan ICM: Circulating immune complexes in inflammatory bowel disease. *Clin Exp Immunol* 14:219, 1973.

Korsmeyer SJ, Williams RC Jr, Wilson ID, et al: Lymphocytotoxic antibody in inflammatory bowel disease. *N Engl J Med* 293:1117, 1975.

Lagercrantz R, Hammarstrom S, Perlmann P, et al: Impaired anamnestic cellular immune response in patients with Crohn's disease. *Gut* 16:854, 1975.

Sachar DB, Taub RN, Brown SM, et al: Impaired lymphocyte responsiveness in inflammatory bowel disease. *Gastroenterology* 64:203, 1973.

Shorter RG, Huizenga KA, ReMine SG, et al: Effects of preliminary incubation of lymphocytes with serum on their cytotoxicity for colonic epithelial cells. *Gastroenterology* 58:843, 1970.

Thayer WR: Crohn's disease: The immune complex disease? *Excerpta Medical International Congress Series* 386:113, 1976.

7 Is Investigation Headed in the Right Direction?

David B. Sachar, MD

I have been charged with a very provocative and challenging question: "Is investigation headed in the right direction?" I shall attempt to respond to that challenge according to the Talmudic tradition in answering a question with a question; in fact, two questions.

The first question is: "Is there a direction in which research is headed?" The second question is: "Can anybody presume to guess which of those directions is the right direction?"

With respect to the first question, I believe we already have the feeling that the answer is really *no*. There is no one direction in which people are going. The reason is all too obvious today: nobody really knows in what direction to look. These are diseases with no definitely known etiology and pathogenesis. Certainly there are diseases where we know the etiology, such as viral hepatitis or alcoholic pancreatitis, but do not fully understand the pathogenesis—how the cause induces the disease. There are other diseases where we understand the pathologenesis, such as knowing that acid has something to do with ulcers, or that cholesterol concentration of bile has something to do with gallstones. With ileitis and colitis we are in the dubious position of having no concept either of etiology or of pathogenesis. Because these are unknown, we really have to look in every direction when we talk about a direction of research. We shall now review some of the principal and promising areas in each of six directions.

The first area where investigators are seeking for an understanding of Crohn's disease has to do with its *pathology*. While there is a concept of the final appearance of Crohn's disease in terms of stenotic, cobblestoned, fat-encased lesions, the early lesions of the disease are being increasingly studied. It is very promising to investigate the tiny aphthoid ulcerations which may be how the disease begins. These early lesions may also provide some clues concerning etiology. One clue is to the luminal origin of the agent that initiates the disease. A second clue may be to study the tiny ulcerations more closely.

Besides studying the early lesion, a second area worth considering is to investigate where in the gastrointestinal tract the disease strikes. As has been pointed out, it can be anywhere from the mouth to the anus. But as we study the distribution of lesions throughout the gastrointestinal tract, we find that, while less than one-fifth of the cases are confined to the colon, two-thirds involve the colon with spillover to the ileocecal valve, thus involving both ileum and colon. Finally, a splinter group attacks other areas like the mouth or esophagus, stomach, duodenum, and anus. This suggests that any hypothesis about the nature of the disease based on the belief it is merely ileitis or a disease that strikes lymphoid-rich areas or areas proximal to sphincters, must take into account the fact that this is a disease of more diffuse targeting. We must remember that two-thirds of the cases spread beyond the ileum.

Perhaps another clue in terms of pathology is the granuloma in Crohn's disease. Does this suggest some kind of impaired hypersensitivity or some type of persisting antigen? However, it is possible that in Crohn's disease a granuloma will not be found in draining lymph nodes unless it is also present in the bowel wall, which is the reverse of the situation in ileocecal tuberculosis where a granuloma may occur in nodes but not necessarily in the bowel wall. This observation may point to the possibility that the disease has a luminal origin and spreads serosally.

A second area to be studied is how the disease behaves. What is the *natural history* of the disease? What lessons can we learn about etiology and pathogenesis from the natural history? One of the first points that we can make is that this disease in some way seems to follow the intestinal stream. Surgeons, gastroenterologists, and pathologists are all familiar with the situation in which an otherwise normal colon — right at the site where a fistula enters it from adjacent diseased ileum — will begin to develop excrescences and nodular granulomatous lesions. With diversion of the intestinal stream these lesions may heal; with reestablishment of intestinal continuity they tend to recur. Thus there may be something in the intestinal stream which is delivering a toxic agent to the bowel wall.

The next area of natural history being studied concerns colitis-related, extraintestinal manifestations.[1] These are very common manifestations, occurring in about one-third of patients with inflammatory bowel disease. They are noted at least twice as commonly in patients who have colonic inflammation as in those in whom inflammation is limited to the small bowel. Furthermore, approximately one-third of patients with any of these manifestations will have yet another one. What these extraintestinal manifestations may be trying to tell us, at least in the case of the peripheral joint and skin manifestations, is that there is some type of circulating immunomicrobiologic factor, perhaps immune complexes. Another lesson these manifestations might be trying to give us with respect to ankylosing spondylitis, sacroiliitis, and anterior uveitis, is that there also may be a genetic factor in the predisposition to these diseases transferred by the HLA antigen B27.

When we are studying natural history, another important area of research that cannot be ignored is the issue of cancer. The problem of cancer risk, to some extent in Crohn's disease and especially in ulcerative colitis, is a major issue that requires research.[2] As we are following patients longer, using actuarial techniques, we are beginning to find for the first time that the risk of cancer development in ulcerative colitis is not limited to patients with universal or pan-colitis. When patients are followed long enough, into the 20- and 30-year range, one finds the development of cancer in patients with left-sided colitis. The incidence of cancer in left-sided colitis virtually parallels that in universal disease, but with the curve shifted about ten years to the right. The magnitude of this problem has not been fully appreciated because of the inadequate period of follow-up. Perhaps no patient with any significant degree of colitis should really consider himself immune to the need for cancer surveillance.

While it was formerly taught that anybody who develops colitis early in life has an increased risk of cancer, we now find there is actually no increase in cancer risk with earlier age of onset. In other words, we cannot show an increased cancer risk in childhood-onset cases independent of their customarily longer periods of follow-up. Furthermore, we now find that the mortality in cases of cancer associated with ulcerative colitis is no greater than that of cancer of the colon in the general population. This observation has some important implications for the value of surveillance. It is to be hoped that the search for early warning signs of dysplasia in rectal and colonic biopsies may give advance warning of premalignant potential.

The last area in natural history to be discussed is the problem of recurrence.[3] Clinicians are familiar with the problem of recurrence in Crohn's disease after surgery, but what needs to be appreciated is its quantitative magnitude. If one follows patients long enough, recurrence and even re-operation of Crohn's disease after an initial anastomotic procedure is virtually inevitable. This is because the cause of the disease has obviously not been removed.

The third area of research is *epidemiology and genetics*. First, the incidence and prevalance of Crohn's disease are increasing. The figures for incidence used to be 2 per 100,000 per year; later they became 4 per 100,000 per year; and now the latest incidence for certain areas of the country is 10 to 12 per 100,000 per year. The same kind of striking increase is associated with prevalence. It used to be considered about 40 per 100,000; then 70 per 100,000; and some of the figures now being quoted from high population centers are in the range of 120 or 150 per 100,000. The second point is that the high family incidence has yet to be reliably attributed to either epidemiology or genetics. Schwartz and his associates in Syracuse have reported that in sibling pairs with inflammatory bowel disease, there is complete concordance in both the A and B haplotypes of the HLA antigen complex in about 80% of the cases. Our own studies, however, have not demonstrated increased HLA incidence concordant among siblings with inflammatory bowel disease.

The fourth area of research is that of *immunology*.[4,5] There are many types of autoantibodies associated with this disease but their pathogenetic significance has never been proven. Lymphocytes are cytotoxic to the colonic epithelium, but this cytotoxicity may not be the primary initiating mechanism since the phenomenon disappears with the removal of the target organ. There are also some new data suggesting that the cells responsible for mediating the antibody-induced cellular cytotoxicity may not be present in the intestine. Thus it is still not clear whether lymphocytic cytotoxicity really plays a pathogenetic role. With respect to the matter of impaired cellular immunity, there are continuing controversies, although it is believed that at least one-third of patients with inflammatory bowel disease have impaired cellular immunity by one criterion or another: hyperexpansive lymphocytes, suppressed T cell proportions and absolute counts, and cutaneous anergy. Indeed, we have found cutaneous anergy to dinitrochlorobenzene in about 50% of patients with ulcerative colitis and 70% with Crohn's disease. We have also studied their first-degree relatives and their spouses and find no increased incidence of cutaneous anergy. What is most interesting is that when the target organ in ulcerative colitis is removed, skin reactivity appears to revert to normal, whereas in Crohn's disease it remains unchanged.[6] Thus when you take out the target organ you have not eradicated the disease in Crohn's disease, whereas you have in ulcerative colitis.

The fifth area of research is concerned with *therapy*. Surgical therapy may be a bright spot on the horizon. Until now, surgeons have been playing the "numbers game," namely, seeing how often Crohn's disease recurs, how many patients get recurrences, and who does and who does not. What has been overlooked is the matter of whether the patient does or does not suffer recurrences, as well as the quality of his life. How do patients feel about having been operated on, whether they have ileostomies or not, whether they have recurrences or not? In following our patients who underwent primary elective surgery for Crohn's disease five to ten years before, we found that in every area of psychological function—social function, sexual activity, body image, job performance, recreation, etc—there was a highly significant improvement, even in the presence of an ileostomy or disease recurrence, and even in the presence of subsequent re-operation. This matter should be something to be studied more in the future: the issue of the quality of life, and not just the "numbers game."[7]

With regard to the sixth and final area of research, there is still no clear-cut knowledge about *etiology*. The early studies concerning viruses and bacteria were either negative or not reproducible. The phenomenon of granuloma transmission to animals is mostly nonspecific. The experiments are not reproducible. They are not uniform. They are not consistent. Many of them have been shown to be artifacts. The same applies to viruses. Better assay systems are required that can produce these putative viral particles in higher titer—perhaps epithelial cell cultures, or fetal gut organ cultures. Meanwhile, reports of atypical *Mycobacteria* in the tissues of patients with Crohn's disease are unconfirmed. The reports of the cell-wall-deficient *Pseudomonas* forms are intriguing, but there are problems in the reproducibility of those phenomena and in the reproducibility of their serologic manifestations. The possibility of *Chlamydia* being involved is based on only one unconfirmed report.

REFERENCES

1. Greenstein AJ, Janowitz HD, Sachar DB: The extraintestinal complications of Crohn's disease and ulcerative colitis: A study of 700 patients. *Medicine* 55:401–412, 1976.

2. Greenstein AJ, Sachar DB, Smith H, et al: Cancer in universal and left-sided ulcerative colitis: factors influencing risk. *Gastroenterology* 77:290–294, 1979.

3. Greenstein AJ, Sachar DB, Pasternack BS, et al: Reoperations and recurrences in Crohn's colitis and ileocolitis: crude and cumulative rates. *N Engl J Med* 293:685–690, 1975.

4. Strickland RG, Sachar DB: The immunology of inflammatory bowel disease, in

Progress in Gastroenterology, vol. III, ed by GB Jerzy Glass, New York, Grune & Stratton, 1977, pp 821–838.

5. Sachar DB, Auslander MO, Walfish JS: Aetiologic theories of inflammatory bowel disease. *Clin Gastroenterol* (in press).

6. Meyers S, Sachar DB, Taub RN, et al: Significance of anergy to DNCB in inflammatory bowel disease: family and post-operative studies. *Gut* 19:249–252, 1978.

7. Meyers S, Walfish JS, Sachar DB, et al: The quality of life after surgery for Crohn's disease: a psychosocial assessment. *Gastroenterology* 78:1–6, 1980.

8 What is Considered Good Medical Care In Crohn's Disease?

Burton I. Korelitz, MD

Some of the complex problems seen in Crohn's disease are accentuated by late diagnosis. We have reached a point where the disease has become so prevalent that we have to think of it sooner. What are some of the early symptoms that should make us suspicious?

If a patient, particularly a young one, presents with combinations of symptoms such as loose stools plus pallor, or loose stools and weight loss, or frequent intestinal upsets and an extra symptom like rectal pain, Crohn's disease should at least be considered in the differential diagnosis (Table 8-1).

Table 8-1
Symptoms Which Should Arouse Suspicion of Crohn's Disease

Anorexia	Malaise
Loose stools	Awakening at night
Pallor	Weight loss
Rectal pain	Intestinal upsets

Additional symptoms that should more strongly suggest the possibility of Crohn's disease as a diagnosis (Table 8-2) include those mimicking appendicitis which is so much more common than Crohn's disease. If the index of suspicion is high, it might not necessarily prevent an operation, but it will at least give the surgeon time to think about what he will do when he discovers that Crohn's disease is the true diagnosis as opposed to conventional appendicitis. Certainly if fever is combined with loose stools or frequent intestinal upsets or anemia, and the patient then presents with a perirectal abscess or fistula, there should be a high index of suspicion of Crohn's disease leading to a workup including sigmoidoscopy, barium enema, and gastrointestinal and small bowel series which might or might not show the disease more proximally. The entire involvement with Crohn's disease might be limited to the appendix. Anal skin tabs sometimes herald a diagnosis of Crohn's disease, and nothing else might be found for some time to come. Certainly retarded growth and development in a child, particularly when combined with any of the other symptoms, should make the doctor suspicious.

Table 8-2
Conditions Which Confirm or Arouse *High* Suspicion of Crohn's Disease

Appendicitis	Perirectal abscess
Fever	Perirectal fistula
Anemia	Anal skin tabs
Retarded growth and development	

There is a particular problem in pediatric practice where the pediatrician confronts children with diarrhea of all kinds and customarily prescribes an antidiarrheal agent which will often work. Then the episode might be forgotten.

Thus the pediatrician must be astute and know when to proceed with further workup. Once symptoms like those shown in Table 8-3 are noted, especially if they occur in combination with some of those already noted, the diagnosis should then be clear-cut. These are all late symptoms. Fistulae and malabsorption syndromes are obvious. Hemorrhage occurs rarely, but early in the course of the disease it can be massive. Abdominal tenderness and mass, obstruction, and the extraintestinal symptoms should all lead to quick diagnosis. These are all overt symptoms of Crohn's disease and the workup will probably lead to the obvious diagnosis.

Table 8-3
Late Symptoms of Crohn's Disease

Diarrhea	Abdominal tenderness
Fistulae	Abdominal mass
Malabsorption	Obstruction
Hemorrhage	Extraintestinal symptoms

Many clinicians are not enthusiastic about sigmoidoscopy and biopsies in Crohn's disease in contrast to ulcerative colitis. We believe, however, that sigmoidoscopy is of great value in diagnosis and management (Table 8-4). Exudate is found in the lumen, sometimes even when the mucosa looks normal. Often the mucosa looks pasty even though it is nonfriable and without erosions or ulcerations. Congestion or friability may be seen in such cases, just as in ulcerative colitis, or patchy erosions, if the rectum is involved at all, with normal-appearing mucosa between. Occasionally we see gross aphthous lesions. Pseudopolyps may be present, while the rest of the mucosa appears absolutely normal. Rectovaginal fistulae can be seen, and we often find a little polypoid elevation in the anterior wall of the rectum on sigmoidoscopy which is the mouth of the fistula extending into the vagina, while the rest of the mucosa appears absolutely normal.

Table 8-4
Positive Findings on Sigmoidoscopy in Crohn's Disease

Exudate in lumen
Pasty appearance of mucosa
Mucosal congestion or friability
Patchy erosions
Aphthous lesions
Pseudopolyps
Rectovaginal fistula
Anal complications
Strictures

Anal complications are very frequent and sometimes occur by themselves. Strictures may be found, particularly with long-standing symptoms, and the finger or the sigmoidoscope may be passed through a stricture. The mucosa beyond it can seem entirely normal.

Some clinicians feel that the rectal biopsy is a waste of time, but we believe that it is very important. (Table 8-5). It could: 1) confirm the diagnosis of ulcerative colitis or Crohn's disease, 2) differentiate between the two which certainly has great prognostic value with respect to treatment, 3) might reveal inflammation if the mucosa looks normal, 4) enable the biopsy to be used as a fine guide for response to treatment if microscopic inflammation was present initially, and then disappeared coincident with treatment, and 5) provide a more accessible area to examine the disease.

Table 8-5
Value of Rectal Biopsy in Crohn's Disease

Confirmation of diagnosis
Differential diagnosis
Presence of inflammation when sigmoidoscopy is normal
Response to therapy
Index of Crohn's disease activity
Premalignant changes
Research

Premalignant changes are probably much more pertinent to ulcerative colitis, but may also be important in Crohn's disease. Other research projects might yet be conceived in which rectal biopsies will be of value in the general supervision of Crohn's disease (Table 8-6). Certainly when there is active disease, frequent visits are necessary. One of the most important aspects of management of this disease is to try to keep ahead of it, try to determine its course, and be prepared with the next step. Furthermore, some indicators of disease activity must be established for any particular patient, and the clinician must follow these diligently.

Table 8-6
General Supervision of Crohn's Disease

Frequent visits when disease is active

Establishment of indicators of disease activity

Interpretation of symptoms: primary disease vs drugs

Interpretation of symptoms is sometimes very difficult because one must choose between those associated with the primary disease and those due to drug therapy. If an error is made in this area, it can influence the entire life of the patient. In general supervision (Table 8-7), we must be aware of the natural course of the disease. The radiologist prefers a clean colon for a barium enema. Unfortunately this is not always possible in this disease. Since what might be missed are tiny polyps, which are not usually of great consequence, we must prepare the patient with clear liquids and simple enemas but without cathartics. Stool studies for parasites and pathogenic bacteria should be done at least once because amoebae and Giardia are particularly prevalent, and differential diagnosis is difficult at best. Confirmation of the diagnosis, no matter how clear it might seem by sigmoidoscopy or by x-ray, should be made by rectal biopsy. If at all possible there should be tissue diagnosis at least once to avoid missing something unusual or more treatable.

Table 8-7
Other Management Factors

Awareness of natural course

Keeping ahead of the disease

Preparation for x-rays

Stool studies for parasites and pathogenic bacteria

Confirmation of diagnosis

Other supportive measures are required. Diet has only a minor role in the treatment of inflammatory bowel disease. Patients should not be "crippled" with stringent diets. They are already sick enough with their disease. They should in general be permitted to eat what they want. However, if there is a lactase insufficiency, milk and milk products must be eliminated. Partial intestinal obstruction requires modification of the consistency of the diet. Sedatives should be prescribed as needed but in moderation since they can contribute to the development of distention and toxic megacolon. Anticholinergics should never be used for the same reason. They do very little for the disease itself and they certainly predispose to megacolon. Antibiotics have some role following surgery but there is no definite evidence for more than that.

A small bowel tube should be passed in the presence of megacolon and in small bowel obstruction. Elemental diets have a role. Vitamins and minerals should be used according to the judgment of the managing physician. Iron should not be given orally because it is irritating in the active stage of Crohn's disease or ulcerative colitis. If iron is indicated, it should be administered intramuscularly. Antidiarrheals have to be used cautiously because they too can contribute to megacolon. Pain medications require similar considerations. If there is cause for the pain, that cause must be discovered and treated more specifically. Blood transfusions should be used as indicated to facilitate response to medical therapy. A rectal tube is often of value in the presence of a toxic megacolon. Hyperalimentation has more of a role in Crohn's disease than in ulcerative colitis.

Emotional factors have little to do with the cause of the disease in the first place, but they do influence its later course (Figure 8-1). Prolonged stress often precedes the onset. Acute stress, anxiety, or depression, often precede exacerbations but the natural course of the disease is very similar. Furthermore, factors such as problems in the family, sexual dysfunction, and the patient's occupation may influence both prolonged stress and acute stress.

Other factors that may affect the response to drug therapy include the status of intestinal penetration, immunologic aspects, and the site of the disease (Table 8-8). For example, sulfasalazine is more likely to be effective in colonic disease than in small bowel disease. Severity of disease also has an influence on the expected response. The timing of administration of drugs is important in that they might be effective at one time but not at another, depending on the circumstances and what drug has been given before. Management of drug therapy requires skill.

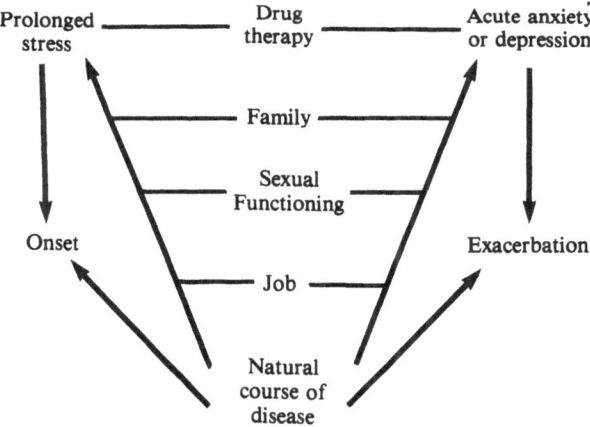

Figure 8-1 Emotional factors: Influence on prognosis.

Table 8-8
Factors Influencing Response to Drug Therapy

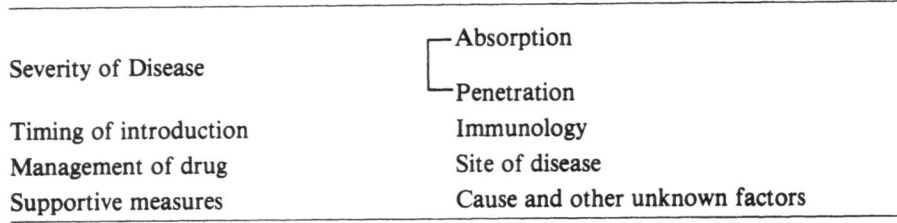

Severity of Disease	┌─ Absorption
	└─ Penetration
Timing of introduction	Immunology
Management of drug	Site of disease
Supportive measures	Cause and other unknown factors

The influence of the rapport between the patient and physician on management might be one of the most important issues (Table 8-9). First, what kind of person is the physician? Is he mature? Is he sensitive to the problem? Does he introduce drug therapy with positivity? What is his background and knowledge about the drugs? How much of his personality is added to it? What about his bias, for or against surgery or for or against the drug? What about his associates, the people with whom he works? Meanwhile, one has a patient who can be independent or dependent on the physician. He may or may not be intelligent. He might resent having the disease and approach it angrily, not ready to accept anything. His emotional reserve and frustration levels are important factors. All of these issues including the course of the disease and the results of management will influence the outcome.

Table 8-9
Rapport Between Patient and Physician

Physician	→ Outcome ←	Patients
	↓	
Maturity	Results of	Independence
Sensitivity	management	Dependence
Positivity	including	Intelligence
Education	drugs	Resentment
Personality	↑	Emotional reserve
Bias	Course of	Frustration
Associations	disease unknown	

With respect to drug therapy, sulfasalazine is still the mainstay (Table 8-10). If it works, it is a boon to long-term management because it may be taken over long periods. If it is effective, it should not be stopped until the cause of the disease is found. If the patient has side effects such as headache, nausea, mild leukopenia, or even a rash, the drug should not be discontinued. It should be given in smaller doses or at different times of the day. If necessary, the patient should be "desensitized" to it. For the really sick patient, steroids are a boon but we have to remember that they are generally not maintenance drugs. Large doses should be given initially to suppress the disease. Then there is some leeway in determining how quickly the drug should be stopped. It can be reintroduced at a later date if necessary.

Table 8-10
Attitude of Physician Toward Drugs: Influence on Prognosis

1. Sulfasalazine: headache, nausea, leukopenia, rash
2. Steroids: dose, maintenance
3. Immunosuppressives: Early complications
   Late complications

9 What is the Role of Immunosuppressive Therapy in Inflammatory Bowel Disease?

Daniel H. Present, MD

There are a number of reasons for using immunosuppressive therapy in inflammatory bowel disease (IBD). First is the chronicity of the problem. The second is that many of the available drugs are not effective. A third reason is the high recurrence rate following surgical removal of the disease. A fourth factor has to do with the varied immunological markers seen in patients with IBD. We see arthritis, erythema nodosum, and numerous in vivo and in vitro immunological abnormalities. All of these suggest that this immune reaction is an impartial factor in perpetuating this disease.

What are the immunosuppressive drugs that have been used to treat inflammatory bowel disease? Azathioprine and mercaptopurine are the drugs that have been used predominantly. They are purine analogs. Other drugs such as the nitrogen mustards and cyclophosphamide were used formerly. Steroids also have an immunosuppressive effect. The mechanism of action of some of these agents has been questioned; are they antiinflammatory as well as immunosuppressive? Both azathioprine and mercaptopurine have been shown to have some antiinflammatory action.

Azathioprine is an S-substituted 6-mercaptopurine. It is an imidazole derivative, and in the first step of the degradation process azathioprine is broken down to

43

6-mercaptopurine in vivo. It is then oxidized by xanthine oxidase into active nucleotides. These interfere with nucleic acid synthesis, and this mechanism is a prerequisite to the ultimate effect. As far as is known, mercaptopurine and azathioprine are essentially almost identical. However, this has not been tested clinically in humans. Using in vitro techniques, azathioprine appears to be more effective, whereas in animal in vivo studies, there are subtle differences depending on how the drug is administered.

There are a number of uncontrolled studies in the literature using immunosuppressives in ulcerative colitis. Scientists tend to dismiss these and call them "anecdotal." However, when one looks at the total number of anecdotal studies, you may come to surprising conclusions. One of the early papers on immunosuppressive therapy of ulcerative colitis was that of Bean in 1966. He used mercaptopurine in six patients and described miraculous improvements. When he stopped the drugs the disease was exacerbated. This paper was followed by numerous others. Bowen reported that eight of ten ulcerative colitis patients improved, and one case of pyoderma gangrenosum healed completely. McKay had nine of twelve patients improved. He found that if he used azathioprine together with steroids a better response was noted than if steroids alone were used. He suggested using both drugs followed by azathioprine alone. Theodore had improvement in four of seven; however, he had one death with sepsis. When my colleagues and I first started using mercaptopurine, we gave much higher dosages. With lower doses, the patient takes a longer time to respond, but there is not the same toxicity as with the higher doses. Jones described nine of ten patients as being improved, and Korelitz and Wisch used this drug predominantly in children and found excellent responses to it.

A review of the literature up to 1972 indicated a response rate of 80% in ulcerative colitis. However, there are only three controlled studies in the world literature. The first report in 1972 by Truelove noted that azathioprine did not help in an acute attack of ulcerative colitis, nor did it help in maintenance of remission. But, when the patients were relapsing in second and third attacks, the drug seemed to work. However, this was not statistically significant. The next study was from the Chicago group of Rosenberg and Kirsner. They found that immunosuppressives statistically permitted a decreased steroid dosage. They did not show a significant response in healing. They also demonstrated that when discontinuing the azathioprine, the relapse rate was higher than with a placebo.

Patterson, who studied 20 patients (not on steroids) found that azathioprine gave results equal to sulfasalazine. Since it is known that the latter is effective in ulcerative colitis, this study demonstrated that immunosuppressives are effective. Thus there are three controlled studies showing statistical effectiveness, one allowing smaller doses of steroids, and the final paper suggesting effectiveness in later exacerbations (not statistically significant).

There has yet to be a large-scale definitive study of immunosuppressives in ulcerative colitis. My personal experience with immunosuppressives in ulcerative colitis is limited to 15 patients. Seven patients had complete remission, with partial improvement in five. One patient was allergic to the drug.

What are the indications for using immunosuppressives in ulcerative colitis? Certainly, not in acute fulminating colitis. These drugs have a delayed onset of action, and are too dangerous in the acutely ill patient. There is a strong indication for their use in a patient who is on long-term steroid therapy or is intolerant to steroids. If you have a patient who needs high dosages of steroids or is cushingoid, these drugs will certainly help, at least in lowering the steroid dose.

Immunosuppressives should be used prior to surgery in the patient who has had colitis for only a short time. There is little indication for their use in the patient who has had the illness for 10 to 15 years, and in whom one is concerned about the development of a carcinoma. But for the patient who has had the illness for only one to two years, and has not been controlled with steroids, these drugs may be tried before surgery. In this selected group, my personal experience has been a 50% remission rate. There are not enough data in the literature to show that these drugs are effective as a long-term maintenance medication in ulcerative colitis.

What are the risks to be considered? Specific toxicity will be discussed later, but the side effects are not excessive. It is my impression that the reason why these drugs have not been used in long-term studies is the fear of causing neoplasia. Since ulcerative colitis has a risk of complicating cancer of the colon, it is ethically very difficult to start this group of patients on suspected carcinogenic drugs.

The first study of Crohn's disease in 1965 used nitrogen mustard – and improvement was noted in 9 of 13 patients. Even fistulae were demonstrated to close. In 1966 the first paper by Brooke reported six of six responding to azathioprine. A more extensive study noted that 19 of 24 improved with closing of the fistula. Nine of nine improved in Drucker's study. He used smaller doses and showed slower responses in all patients. Avery-Jones demonstrated four of ten with remarkable improvement, and Patterson 10 of 15 with nine remissions.

A review of the medical literature up to 1972 shows that 70 of 97 Crohn's disease patients responded favorably. In a study by Brooke in 1976, azathioprine was compared with steroids in Crohn's disease. The response rate was 64% with azathioprine and 75% with steroids. He found that steroids were ineffective with fistulae and masses, and azathioprine was most beneficial with fistulae and colonic disease.

A review of controlled trials shows that there are now eight in the literature, including ours. The first controlled study consisted of 15 patients using a two-month crossover technique. There was no statistically significant improvement. This was followed by another report evaluating 22 patients for a period of six months. There was a statistically significant advantage of using azathioprine in maintaining remissions. A more recent study by O'Donahue also shows that azathioprine will maintain patients in remission once it has been produced with other drugs. Watson in 1974 found no advantage to maintaining remission. He evaluated 11 patients and, despite his negative findings, he noted that the patients felt better while they were on the active drug. Klein in 1974 found no statistical advantage to the use of immunosuppressive drugs, but noted that only his placebo patients went to surgery. He questioned whether there was a subgroup that did in fact respond. Rosenberg and his colleagues found that one could decrease the steroid dosage over a six-month period of study and they, too, suggested a responding subset. The National Cooperative Crohn's Disease Study found no statistical difference in the response to azathioprine compared to placebo, and no effect in maintaining remissions. The design of the study was very different from ours and this may account for the failure to demonstrate effectiveness.

My colleagues and I studied mercaptopurine in patients who were treatment failures with all other drugs. All patients had not responded to steroids, sulfasalazine, and antibiotics. We saw over 700 patients and entered 83 in the study. Fourteen were given the drug without being part of the study. Only 10% of our patients actually entered the study. This suggests that 90% can be controlled with other medications. It is important to remember that mercaptopurine is probably not an initial drug of choice. The age and sex of our patients are typical of all other studies. Patients had been ill for a mean of 8.3 years, and 73 operations were performed earlier in 47 patients, demonstrating that this is a chronically ill group. We used small doses (mean dose 1½ mg/kg) for treatment as well as for maintenance. The doses were based on the leukocyte and platelet counts.

A difference between our study and the NCCDS is that if a patient were on steroids, or sulfasalazine, or both, they were randomized to placebo or the drug and maintained on their initial drug during the first part of the study. Our criteria for response was the elimination of symptoms and signs, healing of fistulae (a strong objective criterion), and discontinuation of steroids while maintaining the patient in a good clinical state. There were two groups, crossover and noncrossover. Thirty-nine patients received both drugs, and the crossover occurred after a one-year period. Patients received the placebo for one year, then the drug for one year, or vice versa. In this group, ten failed in both years, whereas 29 improved in one of the two years. An analysis of those 29 patients showed that 26 were on mercaptopurine, and only three were on placebo. The P value has marked statistical significance. The response rate to mercaptopurine was 66.6% (approximately that of the uncontrolled "anecdotal" literature). The placebo response was 7.7%. In the noncrossover group, we had 33 patients. Of the 19 responders, 15 were on mercaptopurine and four were on placebo. The P value was again statistically significant. Fistulae closed in ten patients. Nine of the ten were on the immunosuppressive, and one was on placebo. Another ten improved, of whom seven were on the immunosuppressive and three were on the placebo. The total healing rate was approximately 30%. We discontinued steroids while maintaining the patient in good condition clinically in 52% of cases; steroids were reduced in another 15%. Therefore, three of four patients could either stop or reduce their steroids.

An important factor is the time required to respond to the study drug. In one month we had only 10% responders, in two months 50%, and in three months 68%. It took one-third of the patients more than three months to respond. If we correlate this with the NCCDS in which a patient was randomized to one drug and taken off all others, and the study lasted for only four months, 20% to 25% of the responders would have been missed. The important factor is that the effect is slow in onset, and steroids or sulfasalazine or both must be maintained. After three to four months an attempt may be made to reduce the steroid dosage and often discontinue the drug.

In conclusion, we found that mercaptopurine was effective as compared to placebo both in the crossover and noncrossover groups. It was effective in reducing and discontinuing steroids, and the response was delayed in the closure of fistulae. There were no deaths in the study group nor during the 10-year period since initiating the study.

Twenty patients were maintained on the drug once they had improved. Thirty-two stopped it after improvement, and of those, 18 were ultimately restarted on mercaptopurine. The drug was discontinued primarily for crossover or because the patient opted to stop the drug after completion of the two-year study. Of the 20 patients who continued on the drug, 15% showed further improvement and 80% maintained improvement. The mean duration of this follow-up is now three years, with a range of up to five years. Only 5% relapsed. On the other hand, when we discontinued the drug, one continued to improve, five maintained improvement, and 26 (81%) relapsed. The time until relapse was similar to the time until improvement, namely, very slowly over a period of months. The patients improved again when the drug was restarted, with a more rapid response.

There was a somewhat better response to mercaptopurine in ileocolitis than in Crohn's disease limited to the ileum or colon. The degree of response seemed to be better with colonic cases.

With respect to toxicity, we had two patients who developed severe bone marrow suppression. These occurred early in the study. There have been no cases of this type recently, due at least in part to increased hematologic observation. To use this drug properly, one should have the assistance of a hematologist who has had experience with it. We had two patients in the study with allergic fever, and have seen a number of others since the study was completed. There was one patient with pancreatitis and the NCCDS has had two or three. If recognized early, there is no problem in managing pancreatitis since it responds to discontinuation of the drug. Nausea has been a frequent concomitant, usually not requiring stopping the drug. We had one patient who developed osteomyelitis while on high-dose steroids. This was more likely due to the long-term administration of steroids rather than to mercaptopurine. Late complications have included one patient with hepatitis (not believed to be due to the drug), one with fever of unknown origin, and one with Q fever which was controlled after she started on a trip to Australia. We have had one patient who was subsequently found to have an islet cell carcinoma of the pancreas. He received the drug for one year with a good response. Whether this is a drug-related reaction or not is unknown. We have had no deaths in either the long- or short-term studies.

One patient had a fistula extending from the colon into the stomach, with vomiting of fecal material. The barium enema of 1977 showed filling of the colon, stomach, and small bowel. The patient was started on immunosuppressives, and x-rays taken in April 1978 did not show any fistula.

What are the indications for the use of immunosuppressives in Crohn's disease? Certainly not in acute fulminating disease. These drugs take two to five months or longer to be effective and, therefore, should not be used in acute situations. They should definitely be used in patients on chronic steroid therapy or with intolerance to steroids. This is a prime indication. They are also indicated prior to surgery, especially with predominantly colonic disease, although they can be used in all areas of involvement. The presence of a fistula is probably a prime indication. The data in the literature seem to indicate that mercaptopurine should be used for maintenance therapy. Our study seems to confirm that if the patient is maintained on the drug, improvement continues.

The final consideration concerns neoplasia. Essentially, there have been some chromosomal changes demonstrated in vitro and in vivo. Teratogenesis has been demonstrated in animals but not in humans and, thus far, the children born of transplant patients who received this drug have not shown any teratogenic effect. The data on carcinogenesis in animals vary, depending on the species of animal used. Certainly we have seen a high incidence of lymphomas in transplant patients, but the animal studies seem to indicate that this is due to the antigenic stimulus of the kidney itself. In autoimmune diseases, mercaptopurine has been now used for 10 to 15 years, and thus far no one has demonstrated an increased incidence of carcinoma. For the present at least, there is strong justification for using this drug in Crohn's disease.

BIBLIOGRAPHY

Bean RHD: Treatment of ulcerative colitis with antimetabolites. *Br Med J* 1:1081–1084, 1966.

Bowen GE, Irons GV Jr, Rhodes JB, et al: Early experiences with azathioprine in ulcerative colitis: A note of caution. *JAMA* 195:460–464, 1966.

Brooke BN, Hoffmann DC, Swarbrick ET: Azathioprine for Crohn's disease. *Lancet* 2:612–614, 1975.

Brooke BN, Javett SL, Davison OW: Further experience with azathioprine for Crohn's disease. *Lancet* 2:1050–1053, 1973.

Brown CH, Achkar E: Azathioprine therapy for inflammatory bowel disease: A preliminary report. *Am J Gastroenterol* 54:363–377, 1970.

Drucker WR, Jeejeebhoy KN: Azathioprine: An adjunct to surgical therapy of granulomatous enteritis. *Ann Surg* 172:618–625, 1970.

Jewell DP, Truelove SC: Azathioprine in ulcerative colitis: An interim report on a controlled therapeutic trial. *Br Med J* 1:709–712, 1972.

Jewell DP, Truelove SC: Azathioprine in ulcerative colitis: Final report on controlled therapeutic trial. *Br Med J* 4:627–630, 1974.

Klein M, Binder JH, Mitchell M, et al: Treatment of Crohn's disease with azathioprine: A controlled evaluation. *Gastroenterology* 66:916–922, 1974.

Korelitz BI, Glass JL, Wisch N: Long-term immunosuppressive therapy of ulcerative colitis: Continuation of a personal series. *Am J Dig Dis* 18:317–322, 1973.

Korelitz BI, Glass JL, Wisch N: Long term observations of children with ulcerative colitis treated with an immunosuppressive (6-mercaptopurine) (abstract). *Gastroenterology* 72:1083, 1977.

Korelitz BI, Wisch N: Long term therapy of ulcerative colitis with 6-mercaptopurine: A personal series. *Am J Dig Dis* 17:111–118, 1972.

Lennard-Jones JE, Williams CB: Azathioprine in the treatment of Crohn's disease. *Proc R Soc Med* 65:291–293, 1972.

McKay IR, Wall AJ, Goldstein G: Response to azathioprine in ulcerative colitis: Report of 7 cases. *J Dig Dis* 11:536–545, 1966.

Patterson JF, Norton RA, Schwartz RS: Azathioprine treatment of ulcerative colitis, granulomatous colitis and regional enteritis. *Am J Dig Dis* 16:327–332, 1971.

Present DH, Wisch N, Glass JL, et al: The efficacy of immunosuppressive therapy in Crohn's disease: A randomized long-term double-blind study (abstract). *Gastroenterology* 72:1114, 1977.

Present DH, Korelitz BI, Wisch N, et al: Treatment of Crohn's disease with 6-mercaptopurine. *N Engl J Med* 302:981–987, 1980.

Rhodes J, Bainton D, Beck P, et al: Controlled trial of azathioprine in Crohn's disease. *Lancet* 2:1273–1276, 1971.

Rosenberg JL, Levin B, Wall AJ, et al: A controlled trial of azathioprine in Crohn's disease. *Am J Dig Dis* 20:721–726, 1975.

Rosenberg JL, Wall AJ, Levin B, et al: A controlled trial of azathioprine in the management of chronic ulcerative colitis. *Gastroenterology* 69:96–99, 1975.

Sachar DB, Present DH: Immunotherapy in inflammatory bowel disease. *Med J North Am* 62:173–183, 1978.

Singleton JW: National Cooperative Crohn's Disease Study (NCCDS): Preliminary results of Part I (abstract). *Gastroenterology* 70:938, 1976.

Strickland RC, Sachar DB: The immunology in inflammatory bowel disease. In Glass GBJ (ed): *Progress in Gastroenterology,* vol 3. New York, Grune & Stratton, 1977.

Theodor E, Gilon E, Waks U: Treatment of ulcerative colitis with azathioprine. *Br Med J* 4:741–743, 1968.

Watson WC, Bukowsky J: Azathioprine in management of Crohn's disease: A randomized crossover study (abstract). *Gastroenterology* 66:796, 1974.

Willoughby JMT, Kumar PJ, Beckett J, et al: Controlled trial of azathioprine in Crohn's disease. *Lancet* 2:944–947, 1971.

Wisch N, Korelitz BI: Immunosuppressive therapy of ulcerative colitis, ileitis, and granulomatous colitis. *Surg Clin North Am* 52:961–969, 1972.

10 Hematologic Complications of Inflammatory Bowel Disease and its Drug Therapy

Nathaniel Wisch, MD

The most common hematologic complication in inflammatory bowel disease (IBD) is anemia. Of the many causes of anemia, iron deficiency appears to be the most prevalent. This is at times a rather easy diagnosis to make. But frequently, in inflammatory bowel disease, it is not quite as easy as one might think, particularly since patients with chronic inflammatory diseases have hypochromic, microcytic red cells. Their serum iron levels may indeed be low because of the chronic inflammatory states. Unless one finds a clear elevation of the serum iron-binding capacity, one cannot be certain that it is iron deficiency. Unfortunately, in patients with chronic inflammatory states, there is defective protein synthesis and the serum iron-binding capacity may in fact be depressed or normal. As a result the finding of a low serum iron level in that setting makes the diagnosis of iron deficiency uncertain. Most often, this diagnosis cannot be clearly made without bone marrow examination and determination of the iron stores within the bone marrow.

The cause of the iron deficiency generally is blood loss. However, in significant numbers of patients persistent stool examinations for occult blood have been negative. In fact, there have been studies that have utilized radioisotopic techniques to prove the presence of blood loss in patients whose stools have been negative by routine tests. This has been done through radioactive labeling of red cells and subsequent examination of the stools for this radioactive isotope, proving that there can be significant blood loss leading to iron deficiency in the absence of positive stools by routine techniques. Iron absorption, whether there is disease of the small bowel or not, has been clearly shown to be defective in patients with inflammatory bowel disease. For some reason the bowel does not absorb optimum amounts of iron, even in patients with ulcerative colitis. Iron absorption in patients with anemia from other causes is consistently higher than in comparable patients with Crohn's disease or ulcerative colitis.

This brings us to the question of therapy. Obviously, in the presence of defective absorption, oral iron therapy may not be as efficacious as in other causes of iron deficiency. Injectable iron is thus probably the most efficient way of dealing with replacement of the iron stores.

Megaloblastic anemia ranks significantly lower as a cause of anemia in patients with inflammatory bowel disease, but nevertheless represents a significant number of patients. Of the two types of inflammatory bowel disease, megaloblastic anemia is more common in Crohn's disease. Of the two causes of megaloblastosis, folic acid deficiency is far more common than vitamin B_{12} deficiency.

The usual change seen in the red cells in megaloblastic anemia, namely macrocytosis, may be absent because of the tendency toward hypochromia and microcytosis in chronic inflammatory states. Therefore, the search for hypersegmentation of polymorphonuclear cells and examination of the bone marrow for megaloblastic maturation is usually necessary for diagnosis. Unfortunately, many of these patients have combined deficiencies of iron and either folic acid or vitamin B_{12}, so that the usual findings in the peripheral blood of macrocytosis may not be clearly apparent when one looks at the cells or calculates the red cell indices. However, hypersegmented polys still occur, even in the presence of combined deficiency. Then one must rely on the astute technologists reading the slides, or examine the slides yourself for hypersegmentation. Again, bone marrow examination in patients with combined deficiency may not be clearly megaloblastic. Therefore, one may have to resort to the use of specific serum assays for vitamin B_{12} and folic acid.

Concerning the etiology of folic acid deficiency in Crohn's disease, it has not been clearly shown whether jejunal involvement is necessary to impair folic acid absorption. Interestingly, it has been shown in at least two studies that the concomitant administration of sulfasalazine results in decreased absorption of folate. The reason for this is not clear. Another factor in folic acid deficiency is increased tissue utilization because of accelerated turnover of nucleic acids. This occurs not only in inflammatory bowel disease, but in many other chronic inflammatory diseases such as rheumatoid arthritis. Also, the intake of folic acid may be significantly decreased because of anorexia associated with inflammatory bowel disease, as well as dietary restrictions that sometimes are placed on these patients by the physician. With respect to folic acid deficiency in ulcerative colitis, there does appear to be some decreased absorption of folic acid in the small bowel in patients with ulcerative colitis.

Vitamin B_{12} deficiency occurs in Crohn's disease primarily in those patients with disease of the ileum or in those who have had significant resection of the ileum. It also occurs in patients with anatomical abnormalities that lead to overgrowth of bacteria and competition for vitamin B_{12}. Deficiency in ulcerative colitis is practically nonexistent. One should try to be specific as to the cause of megaloblastic macrocytic anemia. One would not want to give folic acid to a patient who may in fact, have a vitamin B_{12} deficiency along with it, or might have a vitamin B_{12} deficiency as the prime cause of megaloblastosis.

Chronic inflammation as a cause of the anemia in inflammatory bowel disease is quite common. There are significant numbers of patients who have chronic anemia without any evidence of a deficiency state as measured by all current parameters. They have increased iron in the bone marrow, and may be normochromic, normocytic, or actually hypochromic and microcytic. These patients presumably have the anemia of chronic disease and no known hematinics will cause any elevation of the hemoglobin. Therapy really revolves around testing the underlying disorder, and transfusion with packed red cells when necessary.

Autoimmune hemolytic anemia occurs with increased frequency in patients with ulcerative colitis. These patients present with the typical findings of hemolytic anemia: rapidly falling hemoglobin, reticulocytosis, spherocytes in the peripheral blood, and a bone marrow with marked erythroid hyperplasia. The hallmark of the diagnosis is the finding of a positive direct Coomb's test demonstrating antibodies attached to the surface of the red cells. The onset of this disease usually has no relationship to the state of the patient's ulcerative colitis. I have seen patients whose ulcerative colitis has been relatively quiescent, who have presented with fulminating hemolytic anemia, as well as patients whose ulcerative colitis had been quite active. They usually respond initially to corticosteroids but, unlike the usual idiopathic autoimmune hemolytic anemia, these patients become resistant to steroids. Steroids almost never can be tapered off completely without exacerbation of the hemolysis, and the patients frequently come to splenectomy as a treatment for this condition. Although splenectomy may be effective, we have seen patients where splenectomy has been ineffective, but the removal of the colon has led to a hematologic remission.

Drug-induced hemolysis is particularly significant in patients with inflammatory bowel disease because of the frequent use of sulfasalazine. Patients with glucose-6-phosphate dehydrogenase deficiency are susceptible to hemolysis when exposed to certain drugs. This enzyme, G6PD, is necessary for the maintenance of the reductive potential of the red cell, prevention of the oxidation of hemoglobin to methemoglobin, and prevention of subsequent denaturation of the hemoglobin molecule with hemolysis in the presence of any oxidizing agent or any drug which has an oxidizing effect. This enzyme is necessary to counteract the oxidizing effect. Sulfasalazine, unfortunately, happens to be one of the agents capable of doing this. Since the degree of hemolysis is dose-related, patients with mild decreases in this enzyme are less susceptible to hemolysis than those with severe enzyme deficiencies. Some patients with the enzyme deficiency can tolerate small doses of sulfasalazine but, as the dose is increased, the patient may suddenly develop hemolysis. Again, some patients may be on a steady dose of sulfasalazine and go along for a significant period of time and then one day they develop hemolysis. Intercurrent infections in patients with glucose-6-phosphate dehydrogenase deficiency can precipitate a hemolytic episode. This occurs in viral infections, bacterial infections, and particularly in hepatitis. It is possible that these patients might have had some subclinical infection which precipitated the hemolytic episode, whereas, prior to that, they apparently had been able to tolerate the drug without overt hemolysis.

The diagnosis is made by finding Heinz bodies in red cells during the first 24 to 36 hours after the acute hemolytic episode. This is demonstrated only with supravital staining, using certain specific stains in a wet preparation. After the first 36 hours, the cells with the Heinz bodies have been removed from the circulation, as have all the cells that have deficient enzyme levels. This makes enzyme assays useless at this time. Several months must elapse until a normal cell population reappears. The aging cells with the deficient enzyme then show low enzyme levels. This is a rather interesting complication of inflammatory bowel disease and occurs with significant frequency.

Agranulocytosis and aplastic anemia have also been reported as complications of sulfasalazine therapy, but unrelated to levels of G6PD.

The complications of immunosuppressive therapy include leukopenia, thrombocytopenia, anemia, hair loss, hepatitis, infections, and gastric intolerance. None is irreversible, with either reduction in dosage or discontinuation of the mercaptopurine.

Malignancy has not been found to be a problem when immunosuppressive agents are used for other than organ transplantation. The role of antigenic stimulation by the transplanted organ, along with the immunosuppressive therapy, probably exerts some combined effect in terms of stimulating tumor growth. Whether there will be an increased number of neoplasms in years to come in patients with inflammatory bowel disease treated with immunosuppressives remains to be seen.

BIBLIOGRAPHY

Beal RW, Skyring AP, McRae J, et al: The anemia of ulcerative colitis. *Gastroenterology* 45:589−602, 1963.

Dyer NH, Child JA, Mollin DL, et al: Anaemia in Crohn's disease. St Bartholemew's Hospital, London. *QJ Med New Series,* XLI, No. 164, October 1972, pp 416–436.

Franklin JL, Rosenberg IH: Impaired folic acid absorption in inflammatory bowel disease: effects of salicylazosulfapyridine (Azulfidine). Section of Gastroenterology, Dept. of Medicine, Pritzker School of Medicine, University of Chicago, Chicago, Ill. *Gastroenterology* Vol 64 (4), April 1973.

Hoffbrand AV, Steward JS, Booth CC, et al: Folate deficiency in Crohn's disease: incidence, pathogenesis, and treatment. *Br Med J* 2:71-75, 1968.

Johns DG, Bertino JR: Folates and megaloblastic anemia: review. *Clin Pharmacol Ther* 6:362-392, 1965.

Ormerod TP: Observations on the incidence and cause of anemia in ulcerative colitis. *Gut* 8:107-114, 1967.

Smith AN, Falconer CWA, Small WP: Malabsorption in Crohn's disease, in Girwood RH, Smith AN (eds): *Malabsorption.* Edinburgh University Press, 1969, pp 282-289.

11 The Role of Hyperalimentation in the Treatment of Crohn's Disease

Richard D. Robbins, MD

Hyperalimentation has been used in a wide variety of surgical and medical problems. In general, the indications for total parenteral nutrition (TPN), which is an important facet of hyperalimentation, are to maintain an adequate nutritional state or improve it in a previously undernourished individual. Its use is indicated only when oral or tube feedings are contraindicated or are inadequate.

Hyperalimentation had its beginnings at least 300 years ago. Christopher Wren, when he finished rebuilding London, introduced ale, wine, and opium into the veins of dogs, using quills and a pig's bladder. Although our experience is not this picturesque, it is nevertheless extensive.

Typical indications for hyperalimentation in gastrointestinal diseases include pancreatitis, peritonitis, and surgical complications, as well as inflammatory bowel disease.

The use of hyperalimentation in patients with inflammatory bowel disease allows total bowel rest, rapid preoperative nutritional repletion, postoperative nutritional support, and management of medical and surgical complications.

Recognizing the patient with inflammatory bowel disease who is in need of nutritional support requires both clinical and biochemical evaluation. Malnutrition, one of the primary indicators in this group of patients, is due to multiple causes. These can be summarized by placing them in four major groups: 1) inadequate intake due to anorexia, pain, and diarrhea; 2) excessive losses exemplified by protein-losing enteropathy, gastrointestinal bleeding, and steatorrhea; 3) malabsorption of protein, carbohydrate, micro- and macrominerals, and vitamins; and 4) increased requirements secondary to fever, fistula, growth, and replenishment of stores. One common cause is aberration in bile salt and vitamin metabolism due to surgical or disease-related short bowel.

Because of the malnutrition, patients with Crohn's disease have impaired response to medical management, impaired healing of surgical wounds, impaired healing of disease-related fistulae, and loss of immunocompetence. Hyperalimentation produces an anabolic state, corrects deficiencies of protein/electrolytes/trace elements/calories and fluids, and restores immunocompetence.

There have been numerous recent studies documenting the value of hyperalimentation of various types in the treatment of inflammatory bowel disease, especially in the treatment of Crohn's disease. It has become clear that the following results can be expected. In disease limited to the small bowel, the effect is pronounced. In the colitis of Crohn's disease the effect is less pronounced in terms of obviating the need for surgery than in the former category. In chronic ulcerative colitis, the response is similar to that in Crohn's colitis, but is less effective in avoiding surgery. Many studies, however, have shown that, although improvement as measured by weight gain, diminished pain, cessation of diarrhea and increased serum albumin, is ordinarily found in these patients, these clinical remissions can be expected to be relatively transitory. Therefore, if nutritional support is seen as total therapy, disappointment is inevitable.

Nutritional support can be used in preparation for surgery, in terms of correcting metabolic and immunologic deficiencies and placing the bowel at rest. With the use of nutritional support, surgical procedures carry less risk, and smoother postoperative courses can be expected with improved wound healing, decreased number and severity of wound infections, and anastomotic dehiscences.

Similarly, preparation for medical management is one of the prime roles of nutritional support. Nutritional support may encourage the closure of fistulae, may obviate the need for surgery and, importantly, may permit new or untried medical modalities such as steroids, ACTH or mercaptopurine to be effective in a well-rested, well-nourished bowel.

Hyperalimentation can be seen as having two basic roles in the treatment of the patient with Crohn's disease: 1) correcting deficiencies with which the patient presents and 2) buying time to attempt different modes of treatment previously unexperienced by the patient. Within "buying time" is the concept that medical and surgical management can be expected to have better results in patients whose nutritional status is normal and whose bowel is at rest. The results of many reported studies support this concept.

The types of nutritional support that we can offer to patients with Crohn's disease are: 1) TPN using central venous catheters, 2) TPN using peripheral catheters (including so-called protein-sparing TPN), and 3) enteral nutrition, using oral or, more commonly, tube feedings of chemically defined (elemental) diets. The last category has become increasingly important for the treatment of patients with inflammatory bowel disease. Nutritional assessment is an important step to determine the extent of malnutrition, as well as the patient's response to nutritional support. Biochemical tests and anthropomorphic measurements are used.

Total parenteral nutrition using the central venous catheter requires a subclavian or jugular catheter placement, a routine of dressing changes, and the use of a continuous pump. This affords a high calorie/nitrogen ratio. However, there is a risk of pneumohydrothorax and the life-threatening risk of sepsis.

Total parenteral nutrition using a peripheral line is useful when the patient is septic or when the central line would be at risk. It is extremely valuable in maintaining a well-nourished patient for a short period when caloric and protein needs are not as great as those in patients requiring central hyperalimentation. Technically, the availability of 10% fat emulsion has made peripheral hyperalimentation an extremely useful modality. There is some controversy over the availability of lipid calories. However, we have been using them for some time with quite excellent results.

Enteral nutrition is indicated when the gut is functional. Some examples might be: postoperatively when intravenous nutrition is not needed, preoperatively when diarrhea is not a problem and there is no obstruction or high output fistulae, and for supplementation.

The use of small caliber, long-lasting feeding tubes has made enteral nutritional support a viable alternative to the parenteral modes. By designing the concentration, rate, and constituents of the diet appropriately, a good response can be expected.

EXAMPLES

1. A 35-year-old female with a five-year history of Crohn's ileocolitis developed gas gangrene of the left buttock as a result of an ischiorectal abscess. She underwent immediate debridement in the operating room. Postoperatively she was given central TPN. Nineteen days later she underwent emergency panproctocolectomy for uncontrollable bleeding. However, she had an uncomplicated postoperative course with hyperalimentation.

2. A 51-year-old female with Crohn's disease who was on steroid therapy, enteral diet, and peripheral IVs, lost almost 30% of her predisease weight, had multiple fistulae, and depressed immune competence. All three problems were corrected with hyperalimentation.

Serious anorectal complications of Crohn's disease may show marked improvement with hyperalimentation. If surgery is necessary, hyperalimentation hastens the postoperative recovery.

3. A 21-year-old female who had a 2½-year history of chronic ulcerative colitis underwent subtotal colectomy, ileorectostomy, and loop ileostomy for perforated toxic megacolon. The postoperative complications included peritonitis, sepsis, intra-abdominal abscess, and sagittal sinus thrombosis. Upon transfer, elemental feedings were begun using a feeding tube. On the 19th day after the beginning of elemental feedings, the patient underwent additional resection. Postoperative nutritional support was continued via the same route and resulted in a rise of her serum albumin from 1.7 to 3.8. The patient was discharged on a regular diet.

4. A 37-year-old man with Crohn's ileocolitis and previous colonic resection underwent a laparotomy with drainage of an intraabdominal abscess. He was admitted with recurrent activity of the primary bowel disease and an enterocutaneous fistula. Therapy included central venous TPN, steroids, sulfasalazine, and nothing by mouth for four to five weeks. Marked improvement occurred, with partial closing of the fistula.

5. A 28-year-old man with a four-year history of Crohn's ileocolitis presented with a severe exacerbation of bowel symptoms, a perirectal abscess, and sepsis. He was treated with peripheral TPN preoperatively, as well as antibiotics, steroids, and surgical drainage

of the rectal abscess. He was maintained on peripheral TPN postoperatively, and had marked improvement.

Although home hyperalimentation is not generally available, it is becoming obvious that this modality will play an important role in the future care of the patient with inflammatory bowel disease who, in spite of medical and surgical treatment, cannot survive on whatever functioning bowel remains. Intravenous home hyperalimentation requires a highly organized backup system similar to that used in renal dialysis. Unlike the dialysis patient, however, the patient on home hyperalimentation does not require expensive and intricate equipment and, as more experience is gained, it should become more useful. Enteral home hyperalimentation is more easily performed. It is of use in a wide variety of problems in patients with Crohn's disease.

In summary, the role of hyperalimentation in Crohn's disease is based on the poor nutritional status of the patient which, if uncorrected, will render ineffective any mode of treatment. Hyperalimentation allows the bowel to be put at rest, while improving the patient's ability to respond to therapy. Without this modality, the therapy can actually aggravate the condition. With nutritional support, especially in cases of small bowel involvement, symptomatic relief in terms of reduced pain and diarrhea, and closing of fistula can be noted in five to ten days.

BIBLIOGRAPHY

Anderson DL, Boyce HW: Use of parenteral nutrition in treatment of advanced regional enteritis. *Am J Dig Dis* 18:8, 1973.

Fischer JE (ed): *Total Parenteral Nutrition,* ed 1. Little, Brown, 1976.

Reilly J, Ryan JA, Strole W, et al: Hyperalimentation in inflammatory bowel disease. *Am J Surg* 131:106, 1976.

Reinhardt GF, De Orio AJ, Kaminski MV: Total parenteral nutrition. *Surg Clin North Am* 57:6, 1977.

Shils ME, Bloch AS, Chernoff R: Liquid formulas for oral and tube feeding. *J Parent & Enter Nut* 1:2.

Vogel CM, Corwin TR, Baue AE: Intravenous hyperalimentation in the treatment of inflammatory diseases of the bowel. *Arch Surg* 108:460, 1974.

12 Inflammatory Bowel Disease in the Elderly

Myron D. Goldberg, MD

Evidence presented by several investigators suggests that the age-specific incidence of ulcerative colitis and possibly granulomatous colitis, follows a bimodal curve. The incidence first peaks between the ages of 20 and 30, then begins to level off, and a second, smaller peak occurs between the ages of 55 and 60. To explain this, two theories have been proposed. One is that two different populations are being affected and that, with increasing age, there is a change in the immunologic defense mechanisms that increases susceptibility to inflammatory bowel disease (IBD). One other theory suggests that the bimodal incidence curve may represent an expression of two entirely different disease processes.

It is not unusual to observe an elderly person who presents with a reactivation of colitis that had its initial onset during the earlier decades of life. On the other hand, there are those patients whose symptoms of colitis appear for the first time after the age of 50 without any prior history of colitis. The proportion of colitis in people beyond the age of 50 as an initial and primary episode is in the range of 15% of reported cases. However, the incidence of inflammatory bowel disease in elderly persons is increasing as a result of better recognition of its clinical characteristics and greater longevity of the population.

At present, there is little evidence that the bimodal age incidence curves represent two different disease processes. Nevertheless, colitis as it occurs in patients over 50 behaves in a sufficiently unique fashion to distinguish it from colitis occurring in younger age groups.

In general, the symptoms and signs of colitis in the elderly are similar to those in younger persons, except for the occasional lack of febrile response to diffuse inflammation. This phenomenon is well-described in older patients with infection. The extracolonic manifestations are similar in older patients, except that pyoderma gangrenosum is uncommon in this age group. The response to medical therapy, on the other hand, is variable and generally poorer than in the young. Colonic stricture formation or narrowing with bowel obstruction is not an uncommon delayed complication, and the overall prognosis is much more grave than in those with the onset during the earlier years of life.

The onset of colitis in the elderly may seem deceptively mild. This may be due to the stoicism of the patient or the presence of a more striking concurrent disease. The disparity between the mildness of the subjective complaints and the degree of pathologic change may be great. The patient's age itself is a factor in delaying prompt and accurate diagnosis. Most authors observe that elderly patients minimize or accept their symptoms. They appear to be poor observers and tend to seek medical attention late. They indulge in cathartic abuse and, when they come to their physician, it is for unrelated diseases, usually referable to the cardiovascular or pulmonary system, so that associated colonic disease is frequently overlooked. In elderly patients a wide variety of associated diseases that are common to this age group often distort or obscure the patient's underlying colitis and delay its recognition. There is a higher prevalence of arteriosclerotic cardiovascular disease, hypertension, and chronic obstructive pulmonary disease, all of which occur with increasing frequency in patients over 50.

In a series of patients observed by Law and his colleagues, the authors stress the high incidence of missed diagnosis. Unlike prior reviews, they noted that results after surgery were acceptable if the correct diagnosis was made preoperatively. They suggest that the reason for the high degree of missed diagnosis was that physicians did not appreciate that the disease can present de novo in this age group. More significantly, perhaps, others failed to utilize sigmoidoscopy or properly interpret sigmoidoscopic findings. A change in bowel habits more often suggested malignancy or diverticular disease rather than colitis, and these were the most frequently incorrect diagnoses.

Several case reports in the early literature refer to "segmental colitis" or ulcerative colitis with sparing of the rectum. Many of these patients were elderly, with disease limited to the left colon and few recurrences after the initial episode. Brant and Boley in several recent reports refer to the high incidence of colonic ischemia in this age group. They suggest that earlier reports of colonic stricture or acute segmental colitis may in fact represent examples of reversible ischemia. Many of these cases may well have represented either Crohn's disease or ischemic colitis. These diagnoses must be strongly suspected in any elderly patient with symptoms of colitis, especially with segmental disease.

With early and accurate diagnosis, a more rational and appropriate therapeutic plan, either surgical or medical, can be instituted and may improve survival.

BIBLIOGRAPHY

Banks BM, Klayman MI: Idiopathic ulcerative colitis beginning after the age of 50. *N Engl J Med* 249:91–96, 1953.

Banks BM, Korelitz BI, Zetzel L: The cause of non-specific ulcerative colitis: review of 20 year experience and late results. *Gastroenterology* 32:983, 1957.

Berkovitz ZI: Ulcerative colitis in older patients. *Gastroenterology* 39:28–33, 1960.

Boley SH, Brandt LJ: *Ischemic Disorders of the Intestine.* Yearbook Medical Publishers Inc, Chicago, 1978, pp 41–58.

Boley SH, et al: Reversible vascular occlusion of the colon. *Surg Gynecol Obstet* 116:53, 1963.

Carrol PT, et al: Chronic ulcerative colitis in elderly patients: problems in diagnosis and treatment. *Dis Colon Rectum* 7:226, 1964.

DeDombal FT, Burch PRJ, et al: The etiology of ulcerative colitis. *Gut* 10:277–284, 1969.

Edwards FC, Truelove SC: The course of prognosis of ulcerative colitis. *Gut* 4:299–315, 1963.

Evans JG, Acheson ED: An epidemiological study of ulcerative colitis and regional enteritis in the Oxford area. *Gut* 6:311, 1965.

Gebbars J, Otto HF: Ulcerative colitis in the elderly. *Lancet* 2:714, 1975.

Law DH, Steinberg H, Sleisenger MH: Ulcerative colitis with onset after the age of fifty. *Gastroenterology* 41:457, 1961.

Rice-Oxley JM, Truelove SC: Ulcerative colitis: course and prognosis. *Lancet* 1:633, 1950.

Rogers BH, et al: Epidemiologic and demographic characteristics of inflammatory bowel disease. *J Chronic Dis* 24:742–773, 1971.

Schwartz S, Boley SJ, et al: Roentgenologic aspects of reversible vascular occlusion of the colon and its relationship to ulcerative colitis. *Radiology* 80:625, 1963.

13 Special Problems of Adolescents with Inflammatory Bowel Disease

Theodore M. Bayless, MD

Crohn's disease is a young person's illness, with 10% of patients noting onset before the age of 15. Three aspects of inflammatory bowel disease (IBD) in adolescents bear emphasis. First, adolescent patients often present with symptoms not referable to the gastrointestinal tract, including fever or joint complaints. Because of these subtle manifestations, the diagnosis may not be made for many months or years.[1] The second point is that in the prepubescent adolescent with Crohn's disease, the weight gain and growth seem to be delayed in almost all patients with active disease.[2] While only 20% will become "stunted," most of the youngsters with Crohn's disease have some delay in weight gain and growth. The third point is that this change in growth and development is very useful, since it provides a goal for therapy in terms of adequately suppressing disease activity.[3] In general, the illness in the adolescent is at a stage suppressible without scarring or complication. After a number of years the disease in the small bowel may eventually become obstructed, but the author's goal in localized ileal disease is to keep the youngster symptom-free for as long as possible, at least through adolescence, and then use surgery for obstruction in the late teens or early twenties.

PREDOMINANCE OF EXTRAINTESTINAL MANIFESTATIONS

In the adolescent, nongastrointestinal manifestations may predominate.[1] The admitting diagnoses in a series of 58 youngsters reflect the prominence of extraintestinal problems (Table 13-1). One-third were admitted with a diagnosis of infectious collagen vascular disease, including rheumatic fever, juvenile rheumatoid arthritis, fever of undetermined origin, or lupus erythematosus. Thus the physician has to have a high index of suspicion for Crohn's disease. Physicians are becoming more aware of this, but teenagers are still being followed as having fever of undetermined origin or arthralgia, in whom Crohn's disease was either not suspected or in whom the initial x-rays were not adequate.

Table 13-1
Diagnosis at Admission in 58 Children and Adolescents with Crohn's Disease*

Diagnosis	%	Number
Infectious or collagen vascular diseases	37	
Rheumatic fever		8
Fever of undetermined origin		7
Juvenile rheumatoid arthritis		3
Lupus erythematosus		2
Urinary tract infection		1
Inflammatory bowel disease	22	
Appendicitis	14	
Perianal disease	5	
Other gastrointestinal diagnoses	15	
Hypopituitarism	2	

*Reprinted from *Pediatrics* 55:866–871, 1975.

This lack of suspicion for Crohn's disease had led to a lag in diagnosis. With ileocolonic involvement it took 16 months until the diagnosis was made. Blacks with Crohn's disease have also often gone undiagnosed because of a low level of suspicion on the part of primary care or emergency room physicians.[4] For example, a young black lady came to the emergency room with a right lower quadrant mass and was thought to have pelvic inflammatory disease. It took three years until the correct diagnosis was established.

ALTERATIONS IN WEIGHT GAIN AND GROWTH

Alterations in weight gain and growth can be detected in most prepubescent adolescents with Crohn's disease.[2] Most healthy youngsters stay within a track on the growth curve. In contrast, most patients with Crohn's disease will have a decreased speed of weight gain and growth even if their symptoms are quite subtle. If untreated, some go on to dwarfism with markedly delayed bone age. In some young patients, one can recognize this change in weight gain for a year or two before any symptoms are recognized. Our experience is that if one knows the height and weight data in a prepubescent patient with Crohn's disease, at least 80% or 85% will have some identifiable alteration of weight gain and growth.[2]

We can also use weight gain and growth data in monitoring therapy. The decrease in speed of weight gain and growth is probably due in large part to a prolonged and subtle decrease in caloric and protein intake. This is probably the major factor. Hyperalimentation and parenteral nutrition studies have shown that nutritional replacement is a key part of therapy. Other factors include mild malabsorption in a minority of patients as well as increased caloric and protein requirements because of the active inflammation and protein loss. The lesions are analogous to a "burn" of the intestine. There are also the increased nutritional needs of puberty. At present there are no major primary hormonal factors that have been recognized. All of these mechanisms cumulatively interfere with the speed of weight gain, growth, and development.

THERAPEUTIC CONSIDERATIONS

There are very few published guidelines to therapy of Crohn's disease in the adolescent. In general, supportive measures are stressed. Most authors recommend adrenal corticosteroids only for incapacitating relapses and generally avoid their long-term use for fear of growth suppression. Sulfasalazine is often given over a long term, and prednisone is used, again briefly, if the youngster relapses. Surgery is usually recommended for intractability, for numerous relapses, or for growth failure. Surgery for growth failure, which will be considered again later, can certainly be helpful if done before puberty. However, the literature describes 30% to 48% recurrence rates soon after surgery in teenagers who have surgery for active disease.

We have used a different approach.[3] We feel that some features in the pathology of Crohn's disease are potentially suppressible, and that others are nonreversible. We believe inflammation, edema, and "young fibrosis" are at least suppressible. Conversely, longstanding fibrosis, stenosis, well-established fistulae, and abscesses are not reversible. The adolescent usually has mainly the suppressible pathologic features. We have tried to suppress the active inflammation for as long as possible during the growth phase of adolescence. In that way the late obstructive complications are not prevented, but there is a marked diminution in morbidity during adolescence. Many patients, especially those with primary terminal ileal disease, can be maintained through this period with very few symptoms and little morbidity. If the activity of Crohn's disease is ever suppressible, then adolescents with the early uncomplicated illness are ideal patients to be evaluated. These prepubescent adolescents have the added marker of speed of weight gain and growth and sexual development that can be followed to determine the effectiveness of therapy.

Our therapeutic plan has been to suppress disease activity completely as long as possible until puberty is complete.[3] When prednisone is used, we seek the smallest effective dose which eventually can be administered on an alternate data basis to avoid linear growth suppression. This approach works in those patients whose disease is primarily confined to the ileum. Those patients who have more extensive disease, such as widespread colitis or jejunoileitis, are not always as effectively treated. The results of therapy on a disease activity rating is shown for 16 patients in Figure 13-1. At the onset of the study, most patients were incapacitated or had severe symptoms requiring medication. After a number of months some had moderate symptoms not requiring antidiarrheal or pain medication, and others had very mild symptoms. By six months, nine were asymptomatic, some with abnormal erythrocyte sedimentation rates, while others had normal laboratory tests. Thus, after a number of months of therapy, marked improvement was noted in many of the patients. We were able to suppress the active illness in most of these young people. At the end of one year, 11 of the 16 were asymptomatic. Only one had to be rehospitalized during the 3½-year average follow-up. Twelve missed no school whatsoever except for physician visits. They were seen at one- and two-month intervals the first year, but after that they were seen an average of 3.5 times a year. The average long-term dosage of prednisone was 0.5 mg/kg/day, and most were on alternate-day therapy within a few months. All of the patients received either sulfasalazine or tetracycline. When given together with prednisone, it was hoped this would allow a lower steroid dosage.

The improved speed of growth and development is best seen on growth charts (Figure 13-2). This girl, with a perianal fistula at age 9, was not diagnosed as Crohn's disease until age 14. She was treated with daily doses of prednisone and sulfasalazine.

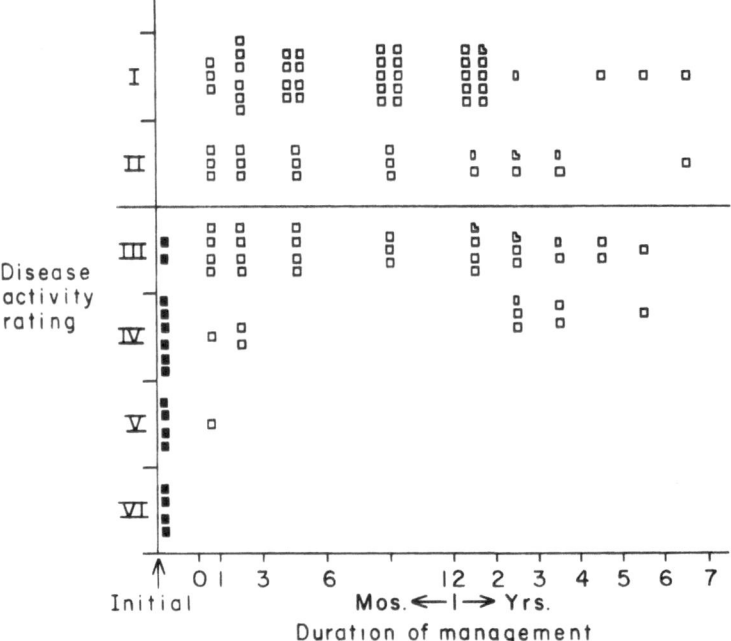

Figure 13-1 Disease activity in adolescent patients with Crohn's disease before and at intervals in months and years during therapy. The definitions of rating scale are: I, asymptomatic with normal laboratory tests; II, asymptomatic with abnormal tests; III, mild symptoms which did not interfere with activities or new physical findings; laboratory tests were usually abnormal; IV, moderate symptoms, occasionally interfering with usual activities; V, severe, requiring symptomatic or antidiarrheal medications; VI, incapacitating symptoms. Each *square* represents one patient experience for the span of that time interval. Incomplete symbols result from changes in status or patient withdrawal during an interval. Thirteen patients were asymptomatic during the 6- to 12-month period. Reprinted from *Gastroenterology* 72:1338–1344, 1977, with permission.

After several months prednisone was gradually tapered to alternate-day therapy. Once alternate-day therapy was achieved, excellent growth and development followed. At age 17, ileal obstruction occurred and she had an ileal right colectomy with anastomosis. She was asymptomatic during the medical therapy period, missed no school, and wasn't hospitalized. She did eventually reach the late scarred stage with very little morbidity.

In patients with localized ileal disease, a gradual tapering to alternate-day from daily prednisone therapy has been accompanied by a growth spurt (Figure 13-3). This patient had a fistula when first seen, but still responded to therapy. The ileum is now quite narrowed and eventually will probably require surgery.

Sulfasalazine alone was used in some patients (Figure 13-4). This has been adequate to suppress mild symptoms and produced good growth results in some patients. Eventually, obstruction occurs in some requiring surgery.

Tetracycline alone has been used in some patients with mild symptoms and localized disease who are allergic to sulfasalazine (Figure 13-5). In general, we have not done as well in terms of growth with extensive disease involvement such as duodenojejunoileitis (Figure 13-6).

Some patients with extensive colonic disease have also been difficult to treat in terms of growth suppression (Figure 13-7). Therapy has included daily prednisone, antibiotics,

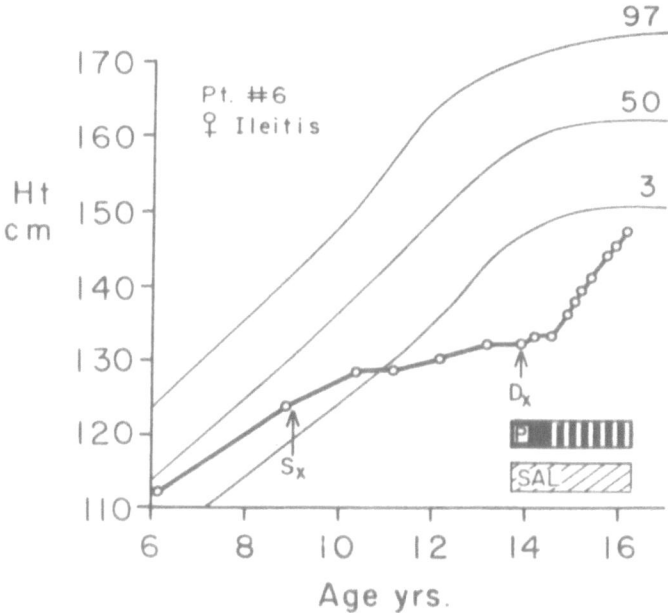

Figure 13-2 Individual growth curves of patients are plotted as height in centimeters vs age in years and superimposed on normal percentile curves of Tanner et al in this and subsequent figures. Sx = symptom onset, Dx = diagnosis, P in *solid* bar = daily prednisone therapy, *striped* bar = alternate-day prednisone therapy, Sal = salicylazosulfapyridine. Patient was referred for evaluation of growth failure. Prolonged gradual tapering was necessary to attain alternate-day therapy. Menarche occurred at age 16. Reprinted from *Gastroenterology* 72:1338–1344, 1977, with permission.

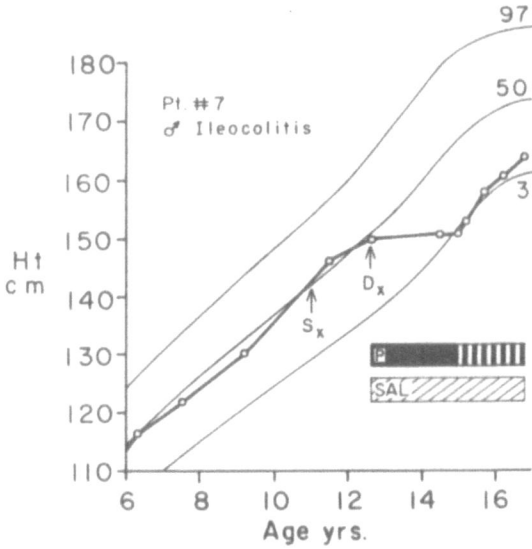

Figure 13-3 Patient was seen in consultation at age 13, but did not enter the series until age 15. Ileocolonic fistulae were present at that time. Prednisone dosage was unchanged but was put on alternate-day basis at age 15. Reprinted from *Gastroenterology* 72:1338–1344, 1977, with permission.

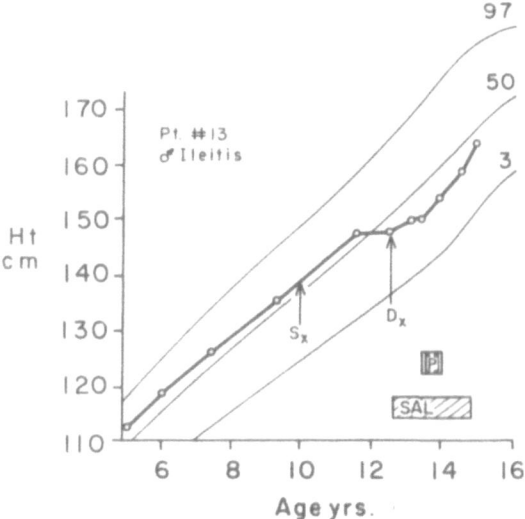

Figure 13-4 Patient had mild episodic abdominal pain and decreased rate of growth when first seen. He has remained asymptomatic with normal laboratory values and unchanged small bowel x-rays since the onset of salicylazosulfapyridine therapy. An eight-month trial of alternate-day steroids was instituted in an effort to influence the speed of growth. Reprinted from *Gastroenterology* 72:1338–1344, 1977, with permission.

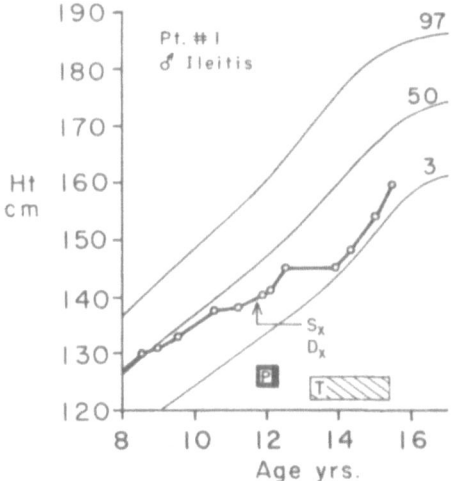

Figure 13-5 Patient underwent exploratory laparotomy without resection at age 11⅓. He was incapacitated with abdominal symptoms when referred for growth failure at age 13. The family, who had consulted with three other medical centers, refused prednisone therapy; patient was allergic to sulfonamides. Management included liberalization of diet and encouragement of protein ingestion as well as long term tetracycline (T) administration. Reprinted from *Gastroenterology* 72:1338–1344, 1977, with permission.

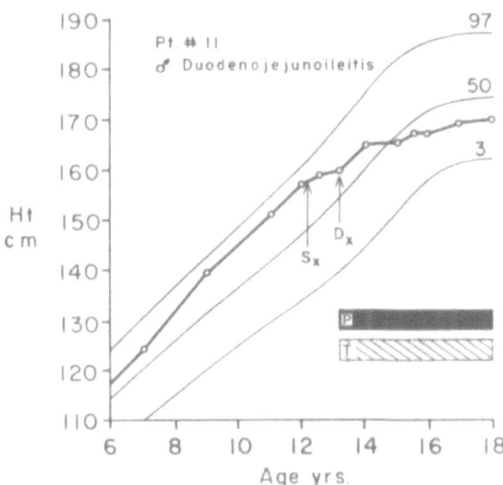

Figure 13-6 Patient presented with fever, anorexia, vomiting, and weight loss. Two trials of alternate-day therapy resulted in symptomatic recurrences. Although he has had occasional mild to moderate symptoms (ratings II or IV), he has pursued a full academic and athletic program, having been state high school champion in both tennis and golf. Although he has not maintained normal growth, height has increased 10 cm during the five years of follow-up. Reprinted from *Gastroenterology* 72:1338–1344, 1977, with permission.

azathioprine, and even parenteral alimentation in some. When the patient and family agree, surgery can result in a growth spurt in some patients, especially if they are still prepubescent. Unfortunately, one cannot guarantee a growth response, but in some patients surgery has been very effective. However, a high recurrence rate after surgery has to dampen one's enthusiasm somewhat.

Most of the patients were able to reach normal stages of puberty. However, those with extensive disease who had to remain on daily prednisone did not develop as soon as their peers.

There were 18 transient, symptomatic recurrences in this group of 16 patients; one in each of eight patients and ten in three patients with duodenojejunoileitis or with extensive colitis. The symptomatic recurrences were associated with a decrease in prednisone dosage in 14 of the 18 episodes. When the disease activity is suppressed, most recurrences occur when the dosage is adjusted. With recurrence we have usually had to revert to daily steroids or raise the daily dose by 10 mg. In general, we could not prevent a recurrence with alternate-day therapy alone.

NUTRITIONAL ASPECTS

It has usually been possible to continue a normal diet, high in protein. We strongly

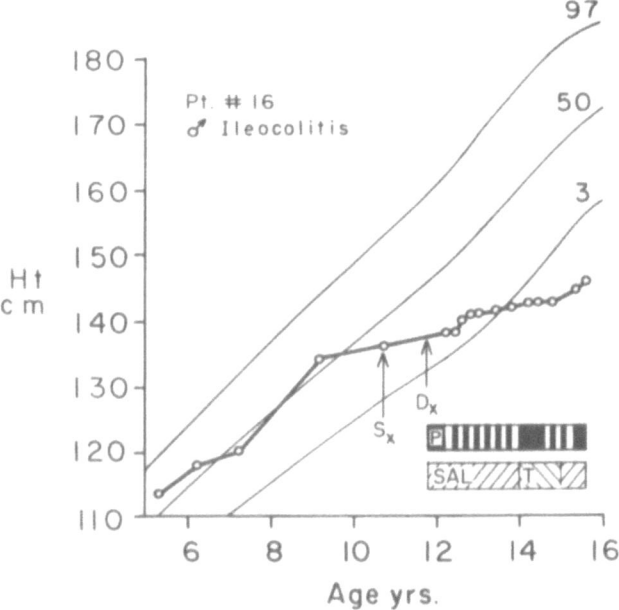

Figure 13-7 Patient remained asymptomatic with normal laboratory values (rating I) for the first two years of alternate-day prednisone therapy. Growth failure was considered an indication of persistent disease activity. Worsening, extension, and probable duodenal disease were confirmed by x-ray study. Parenteral hyperalimentation (3000 calories per day) for four weeks at age 15⅓ years produced only evanescent weight gain. Ileocolonic resection and ileostomy has recently been performed. Reprinted from *Gastroenterology* 72:1338–1344, 1977, with permission.

encourage a very high caloric and protein intake, including nutritional supplements. Studies from the University of Chicago indicate that 80 calories per kilo may be needed to establish weight gain in the sick adolescent.[5] The physician must strongly recommend a very high nutrient intake.

Hyperalimentation has been helpful in some youngsters who are severely growth-retarded.[5,6,7] A course of parenteral alimentation has been associated with a growth spurt in some patients. We have not usually had to employ hyperalimentation because we have been able to prevent severe growth retardation with continual disease activity suppression.

Our goals in therapy for Crohn's disease include making certain that a complication is not present at the outset. Patients with fistulae and obstruction do not respond as well as those with uncomplicated disease. This was confirmed by the National Cooperative Crohn's Disease Study in Adults.[8] An attempt is made to suppress disease activity for long periods and to minimize drug side effects, trying to get adequate growth and development as well as conserve the small bowel. We have attempted to reserve surgery for mechanical obstructive problems if at all possible, and to avoid surgery when the disease is very active or the patient is malnourished. We have used surgery for "a fresh start," ideally for chronic obstruction. We recommend avoiding steroids in the presence of increasing obstruction, for fear of perforation. Lastly, attention should be directed toward the tremendous nutritional needs of these patients. This may require parenteral alimentation or elemental diets.

REFERENCES

1. Burbige EJ, Huang SS, Bayless TM: Clinical manifestations of Crohn's disease in children and adolescents. *Pediatrics* 55:866–871, 1975.

2. Burbige EJ, Huang SS, Bayless TM: Early manifestations of Crohn's disease in adolescents. *Gastroenterology* 66:669, 1974.

3. Whitington PF, Barnes HV, Bayless TM: Medical management of Crohn's disease in adolescence. *Gastroenterology* 72:1338–1344, 1977.

4. Greene CC, Bayless TM: Crohn's disease in the urban Negro. *Gastroenterology* 72:42, 1977.

5. Layden T, Rosenberg J, Nemchausky B, et al: Reversal of growth arrest in adolescents with Crohn's disease after parenteral alimentation. *Gastroenterology* 7:1017–1021, 1976.

6. Kelts DG, Grand RJ, Shen G, et al: Nutritional basis of growth failure in children and adolescents with Crohn's disease. *Gastroenterology* 76:720–728, 1979.

7. Strobel CT, Byrne WJ, Ament ME: Home parenteral nutrition in children with Crohn's disease: an effective management alternative. *Gastroenterology* 77:272–279, 1979.

8. Summers RW, Switz DM, Sessions JT Jr, et al: National cooperative Crohn's disease study: results of drug treatment. *Gastroenterology* 77:847–869, 1979.

PANEL DISCUSSION

Queston: In a young person with a fistula, would you pursue medical therapy or would you go on to surgery?

Dr Bayless: There are two major factors. One is the setting in which the fistula occurred. If the fistula occurred in someone with chronic obstructed disease with a lot of severe cramps beforehand, I would assume that the fistula was decompressing the illness. In that setting I would be looking toward surgery because I think the fistula was just a sign that the patient was obstructed. On the other hand, some fistulae occur in a young person in the presence of very active disease, perhaps because the diseased ileum is lying on another organ with tracking of the inflammation working through the bowel wall. If there is no evidence of perforation or abscess on physical examination, sonography, or radiography, and the patient does not have a high fever or markedly elevated white count, I would consider using an antibiotic. If there were evidence of active disease, I might try a course of steroid therapy many weeks later, in addition to the antibiotic and parenteral alimentation.

Dr Fein: Dr Present, under these same circumstances and with your experience with immunosuppressive drugs, would you be inclined to proceed to immunosuppressive drugs instead? What would you do?

Dr Present: I now have a series of seven patients with fistulae of the bladder whom I have tried to treat medically. You can treat these patients medically with long-term antibiotics and/or sulfasalazine. They can be carried safely for long periods. Thus far, I have followed a patient with intermittent symptoms for six years. Ultimately, many form abscesses and end up with surgical intervention, but I think you can suppress them for years. I have not treated any of these with immunosuppressives. Again, mostly because they have had very localized disease which has responded intermittently to antibiotics or sulfasalazine. When they have gotten sick, it has usually been an abscess resulting in an acutely ill patient in which case immunosuppressives would be contraindicated. It might work, but you should first try a course of antibiotic therapy. You can certainly prolong the situation and not have the patient come to surgery right away.

Dr Korelitz: I have some experience with mercaptopurine for this complication. I have two patients, one with a fistula from the ileum to the bladder and one from the colon to the bladder. Initially, the active disease was suppressed with steroids. We then introduced mercaptopurine and these two patients have remained symptom-free, one for two years, and the other for one year. I feel, therefore, that ileovesical and colonic-vesical fistulae are "former indications" for surgery, but are now only relative indications, and in many cases can be eliminated.

Dr Fein: From these answers you can see that for each patient, you are going to have to tailor the situation. Everybody, I believe, would agree to try a conservative approach first in the hope of controlling the disease. In all of these patients, we have guidelines, and I think you must tailor the treatment for each.

Question: The fear of malpractice suits was mentioned in Dr Korelitz' talk earlier concerning the use of immunosuppressive drugs. I do not think that relates to immunosuppressive drugs alone, but I would like to hear more from Dr Korelitz.

Dr Korelitz: Our double-blind studies are complete. We have no question as to the efficacy of the drug. However, the final document is not yet published. It takes a long time before there is FDA approval. There is no question that gastroenterologists who manage inflammatory bowel disease are using immunosuppressive drugs. At Lenox Hill Hospital we are having permission sheets signed just as if the patient were still in a double-blind study, but we are using immunosuppressives as if they were experimental drugs, even though we do not think of them any longer in this category.

Question: I wonder if the panel would say a few words about rectal steroid therapy and proctosigmoiditis. Do they recommend any sort of "homemade" pharmacy for the patient to save them some money in this type of expensive therapy?

Dr Bayless: I use a lot of rectal steroids for people with proctitis. Let me answer the question two ways. In my own experience, the Cortenema preparation is probably better absorbed systemically than crushed prednisolone. Thus if you want to get some systemic effect, which I sometimes want, or have a patient who refuses to take oral steroids and I want to sneak some in via the rectum, I will prescribe Cortenema because of its systemic absorption. If expense becomes a factor, I use prednisolone and have the patient crush 25 to 30 mg in 1½ or 2 ounces of warm water. This may cost 25 cents a day in contrast to $1.50 or $2 for Cortenema.

Dr Fein: I just wonder if the patients would really be saving that much in the financial cost to the individual.

Dr Bayless: In Baltimore it is $2 a day for a Cortenema. I do not know what it is in New York.

Dr Fein: It is about the same. I think that under the circumstances patients who have this type of disease, even a saving of 50% would not make that much difference where there is the expectation of the symptoms subsiding.

Question: Would Dr Robbins please comment on the cost effectiveness of using total parenteral nutrition (TPN) in inflammatory bowel disease?

Dr Robbins: This has been studied extensively, especially at Harvard. I think it has been demonstrated that in Crohn's disease, as opposed to ulcerative colitis, in the long run it is probably quite cost-effective. In ulcerative colitis, it is a different story, since it becomes a matter of resuscitating the patient with an acute flare-up of the colitis. You are not going to use the hyperalimentation in the same way that you would use it in Crohn's disease. In Crohn's disease, you can really help the patient through the exacerbation. You can probably avoid surgery in many cases, and allow the patient to be treated with various medical modalities. It is certainly life-effective. The studies that Blackburn has done show, I think, that it is cost-effective as well.

The original studies that Dudrick did, both in animals and humans, actually showed closure of fistulae and healing of the perianal region. I remember one striking case that he presented. They were preparing a patient for a total colectomy because of severe universal disease. In the course of preparing the patient nutritionally there was a very marked improvement in the ulcerative colitis, both clinically and radiologically. That patient did not come to colectomy. Of course, that is an unusual situation but I think it certainly has been shown to be of value.

Almost 100% of the patients with Crohn's disease come to surgery at one time or another if they live long enough. It is hard to say that you can avoid surgery forever with any form of treatment. This is something we all have to face. Maybe it is 80%, but a lot of people come to surgery with Crohn's disease. Now, whether or not you use TPN for total treatment, most people today feel that you really cannot just treat the patient with TPN without getting almost immediate relapses. It may be wise to avoid surgery for the time because you temporarily conserve the bowel. I think cost-effectiveness really comes into play more with things like home hyperalimentation, people who have only one foot of bowel left, and they cannot survive without it at home. It costs about $60,000 to $100,000 a year at home, and that is something we are going to have to face in terms of catastrophic insurance.

Dr Present: I think hyperalimentation could be very valuable if you are also using other drugs appropriately. Recently I had a patient with a flare-up of Crohn's disease almost requiring colectomy, but she responded to two to three weeks of hyperalimentation, so much so that we could then start her on immunosuppressives. Now, two or three months later, she is in total remission. I think that with sulfasalazine, steroids, antibiotics, and immunosuppressives, hyperalimentation is an excellent temporary modality for getting the patient into condition to respond once again to one or another of these drugs. I believe that is the indication for TPN, ie, interim therapy.

Dr Korelitz: That is essentially what I believe. I think TPN should be combined with one other approach. The two then go together. I do not ever think of TPN as a treatment form unto itself. Often it gives one a chance to gain a remission and then introduce mercaptopurine for the first time.· Then this drug might be very effective, whereas the reason for which the TPN was used in the first place in itself might not have allowed the introduction of mercaptopurine without the preliminary response to TPN.

Another example concerns surgical resection. There are some patients where surgery is indicated but, particularly in the presence of obstruction, the disease appears too extensive. The TPN then gives us an opportunity to define the disease process more exactly, and it usually is much less than it originally appeared to be. Once that segment is defined, the surgery should be done then, not at a later time.

Question: I would like to ask Dr Wisch about maximum dose levels of mercaptopurine with respect to tolerance, and whether it differs from azathioprine.

Dr Wisch: Initially we used 2.5 mg/kg of mercaptopurine, and we found that this was leading to more problems with interruption of therapy requiring a decrease in the dosage. We have arrived at a dose schedule of approximately 1.5 mg/kg and the majority of patients appear to tolerate this quite well. Some patients still have to have smaller dosages. For some patients who do not respond at that level and if their hematologic status permits, we increase the dose still further. In some of these patients we have been able to get a response at such a higher dosage. The dosage of azathioprine is essentially the same, but I cannot speak from personal experience because we have not been working with azathioprine in our patients.

Question: Dr Robbins, do you use hyperalimentation in Crohn's disease if there is no obstruction or other reason for avoiding the oral route for hyperalimentation?

Dr Robbins: I would choose the enteral route with a tube. I have had only one patient who could drink Vivonex in any significant amount, ie, 2,000 to 3,000 calories a day. That is why we use the tube. We can deliver the right dose to the right place in the bowel. It can be used in any patient who could possibly benefit from the calories and proteins. If they have a colonic fistula, for example, and Vivonex is successfully given and does not produce diarrhea, starting with a half or quarter strength solution at a continuous low rate (30 to 40 ml an hour) into the small bowel and then slowly increased, we can expect that it will be absorbed within 100 cm of the ligament of Treitz. If that is not the case, we are going to have to go to parenteral medication and, depending on the presence of sepsis or the needs of the patient in terms of fat malabsorption, one might choose to use either central or peripheral medication with more or less lipid in the formula. You can design the formula in terms of the patient's needs. We have been using the enteral route more and more with greater and greater success, as we have had more experience with adjusting the dosage levels without producing diarrhea, although sometimes we fail and have to go to a parenteral route.

Question: Should drug therapy be continued during pregnancy?

Dr Korelitz: If the patient is already established on sulfasalazine and becomes pregnant, the drug should be continued. It is tolerated very well during pregnancy. On theoretical grounds, we usually stop it during the last month of pregnancy since some infants may develop kernicterus.

As far as steroids are concerned, if they have to be used during pregnancy, they can be. We hope they will be reduced and even stopped just as if the patient were not pregnant. With respect to immunosuppressives, the patient should not be permitted to conceive in the first place if they are receiving these drugs. Immunosuppressives should be stopped in anticipation of pregnancy. If, however, the patient becomes pregnant unintentionally, then, again on theoretical grounds, an abortion should be performed. In Crohn's disease one should be prepared for exacerbations during the postpartum period. Theoretically, the disease is often ameliorated during pregnancy. In ulcerative colitis, however, if the disease were active at conception, it frequently gets worse.

Question: How long do you generally have to keep adolescents on steroids to be able to induce a remission? Also, please comment on the duration of the course of steroid therapy in adults.

Dr Bayless: Most of my patients are on alternate-day steroids plus an antibiotic. I am uncomfortable leaving someone on daily prednisone for a long time and will add azathioprine if I cannot get the patient onto alternate-day steroids. If I can achieve a remission and growth with sulfasalazine or tetracycline alone during adolescence, I leave the patients on that medication until puberty is completed. If I am using prednisone, I usually leave them on alternate-day therapy through adolescence until they finish their growth spurt. Then we can make individual decisions. The same thing holds true for adults. Most adults have required steroids for several years during the active phase and are on alternate-day prednisone, 20 to 25 mg every other day along with sulfasalazine or tetracycline during the time they need steroids.

Question: Is there any advantage in using intravenous ACTH rather than hydrocortisone, or are they equally effective in equivalent doses?

Dr Present: There is currently a project at Mount Sinai involving more than 50 patients, studying just that problem. The literature is a bit vague on the subject. There was a study at Yale which showed 40 units of ACTH were approximately equal to 100 units of cortisol sodium succinate every eight hours, but we have been using higher doses of ACTH at Mount Sinai. My clinical impression is that ACTH is better.

14 What is the Role of Sigmoidoscopy and Rectal Biopsy in Inflammatory Bowel Disease?

Sheldon C. Sommers, MD

In inflammatory bowel disease, there are really three aspects to sigmoidoscopy and to the rectal biopsy. The first is, what kind of disease, if any, is going to be found in the specimen or by the sigmoidoscopy visually? Not every condition is, of course, either ulcerative or granulomatous colitis. The second use of the sigmoidoscopy and biopsy is to follow the disease as it improves, or re-exacerbates, or whatever its course. The third use is to study the effects of therapies, systemic chemotherapy or steroid therapy, and to gain some knowledge about the pathogenesis and conceivably the cause of the disease.

Some of the salient diseases that have to be excluded before you consider ulcerative or granulomatous colitis are given first. There is a list in Table 14-1 and I will not discuss each one. Sometimes ischemic colitis is very obvious. There is a hemorrhagic necrotizing change in the mucosa and the wall is characteristically thickened. But many cases with biopsies have been considered radiologically and clinically representative of ulcerative colitis. In the specimen, indeed there is ulceration but the essential process is one of ischemic and hemorrhagic infarction, which is succeeded by fibrotic healing. There is hemorrhage, and with our routine trichrome strain in the laboratory, collagen is yellow and muscle is pink. The vessels are thickened and at higher power you see the very narrowed arterioles and small arteries with an inadequate blood supply to keep the mucosa viable (Figure 14-1). The result then, is ischemic necrosis followed by fibrosis. It is a reasonably important differential diagnosis for the pathologist now with the rectal biopsy. Sometimes, there is atheromatous embolism which is the cause of the ischemic colitis. This is almost never recognized before the biopsy.

Table 14-1

Amoebic colitis	Radiation colitis
Amyloidosis	Rectal prolapse syndrome
Balantidial colitis	Salmonellosis-shigellosis
Ischemic colitis	Scleroderma
Pseudomembranous colitis	Venereal colitis

In the colon, we have a possibility of amyloidosis in the vessel walls or in the stroma or both (Figure 14-2). Then there is the unusual condition called rectal prolapse syndrome or the solitary rectal ulcer. The pathologist has to learn to recognize smooth muscle coming up into the lamina propria in cases sometimes initially thought to be proctitis or ulcerative colitis (Figure 14-3). Dr Waye pointed out the little undermined ulcers at colonoscopy that are supposed to suggest amoebic colitis. Here is a biopsy in which the tissue really did not show anything abnormal. The pathologist who examined it did not pay much attention to this material. He thought his duty was to examine the tissue and call it nonspecific chronic inflammation. If he had only looked out, he would have seen

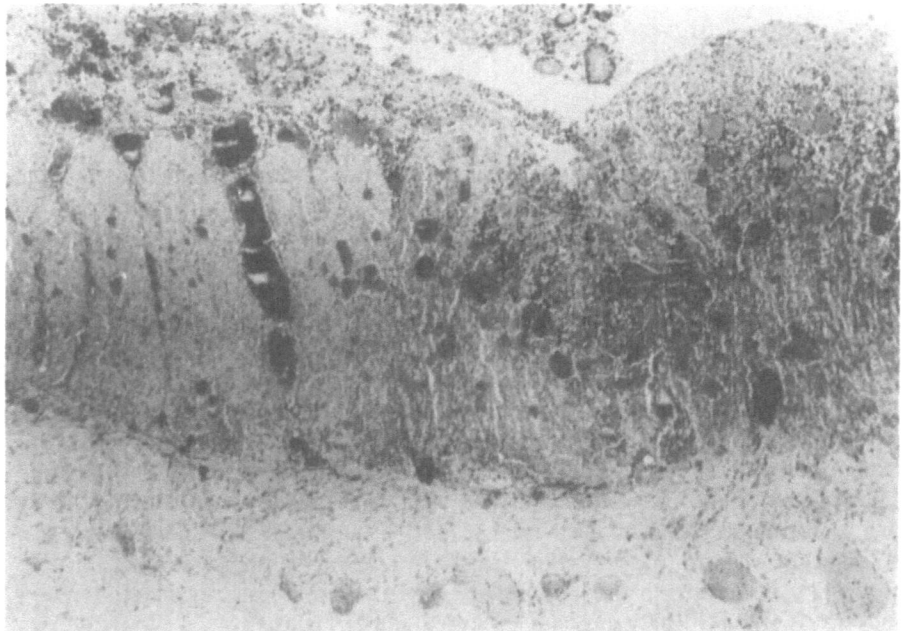

Figure 14-1 Ischemic colitis has ulceration, hemorrhage mild leukocytic infiltration of mucosa and narrowed small arteries. × 100, HPS.

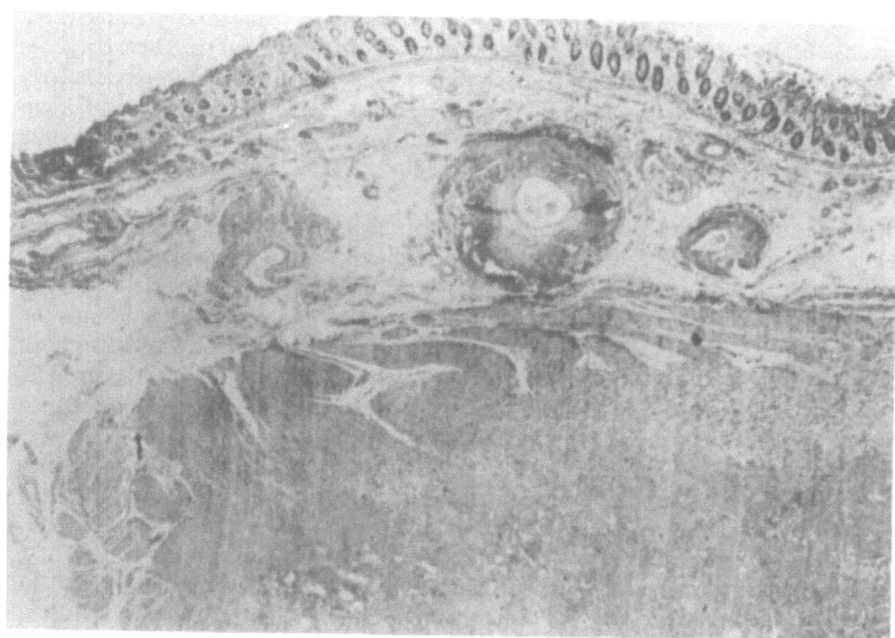

Figure 14-2 Colonic amyloidosis here has notably affected the submucosal arteries but spared the muscularis. × 100, H&E.

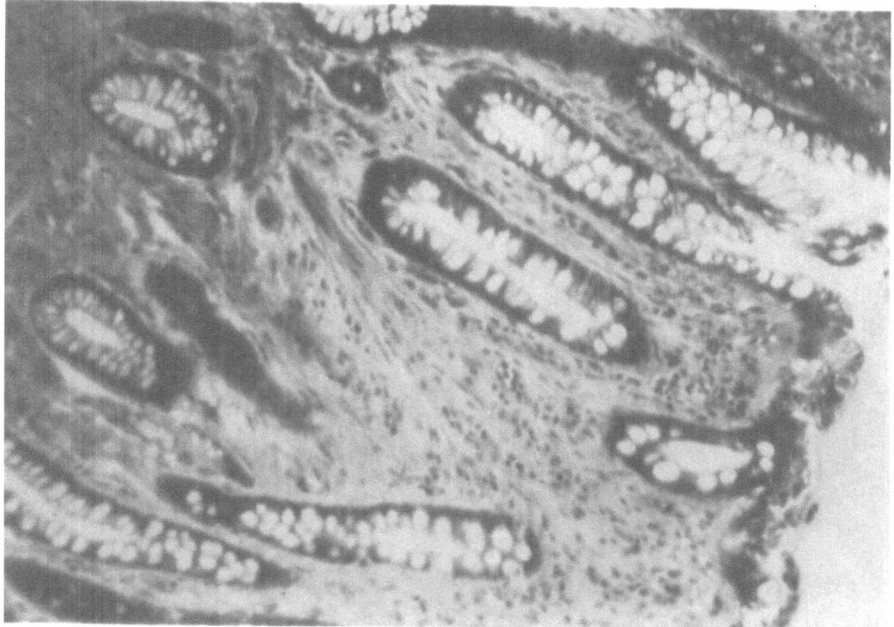

Figure 14-3 In so-called solitary rectal ulcer plump spindle cells that represent smooth muscle permeate the mucosa. × 250, HPS.

thousands of amoebae (Figure 14-4). Unfortunately, this case came to colectomy with a diagnosis of ulcerative colitis, and it was a severe case of amoebic colitis. There is a series in the Archives of Internal Medicine from Philadelphia where every test preoperatively was negative for amebiasis, but that is what it proved to be when there was a sufficient specimen to examine many sections. For the pathologist, I think the major differential diagnosis in this country right now is between amoebic colitis and either ulcerative or granulomatous colitis.

So much then for some of the infectious, degenerative and other diseases that may be clinically and radiologically confused with granulomatous or ulcerative colitis before biopsy. Now to illustrate the fact that if the pathologist wants to pick up lesions nowadays, he has to look at every one of multiple serial sections which may be only the size of a pinhead (Figure 14-5). In this particular case, there were 128 serial sections examined. If the pathologist simply looks at a couple of them, he will miss the small lesions which are diagnosable and which make it possible to find Crohn's disease or ulcerative colitis or some other specific diagnostic entity.

We come next to ulcerative colitis, which is left after all the more specific diseases have been considered and excluded. Sometimes it is easy to recognize because there are practically no mucous goblet cells. There is notable inflammation of the lamina propria, there is an ulcer and there is a crypt abscess full of neutrophils, which is typical of a medical student type diagnostic biopsy (Figure 14-6). You cannot expect that in any individual case. You have to look for somewhat more subtle criteria. One of them is that neutrophils, polymorphonuclears, will overrun the epithelium of the crypts. That is seen

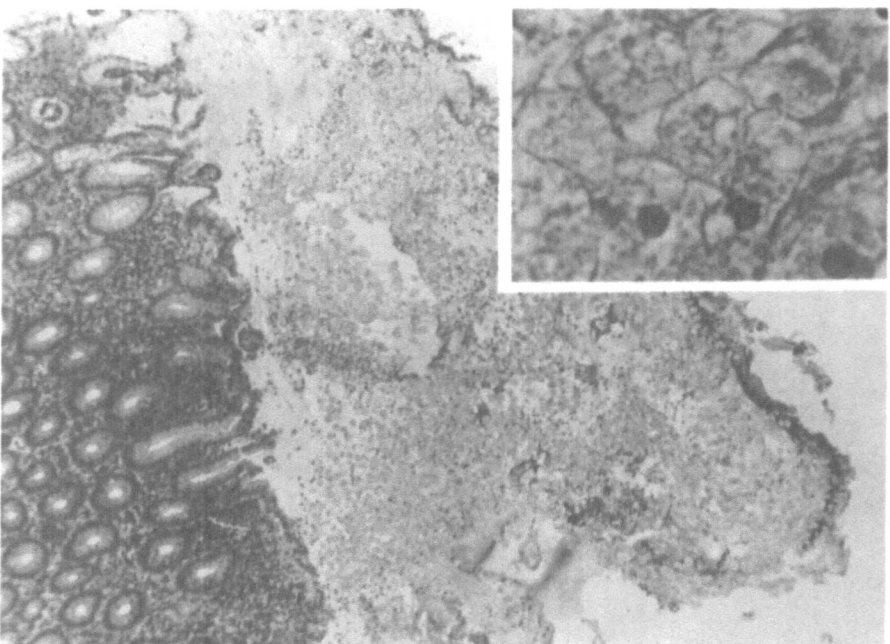

Figure 14-4 Sigmoid biopsy of mucosa showed only nonspecific inflammation. The surface cloud is a myriad of amebae, some of which are demonstrated enlarged in the inset. × 100, inset × 500, HPS.

only in nonspecific ulcerative colitis and to some extent in shigellosis, but the severity of the inflammation and the diffuseness are not nearly so great in shigellosis. It is possible to have a pseudopolyp come as part of the rectal or sigmoidoscopic biopsy. This is just

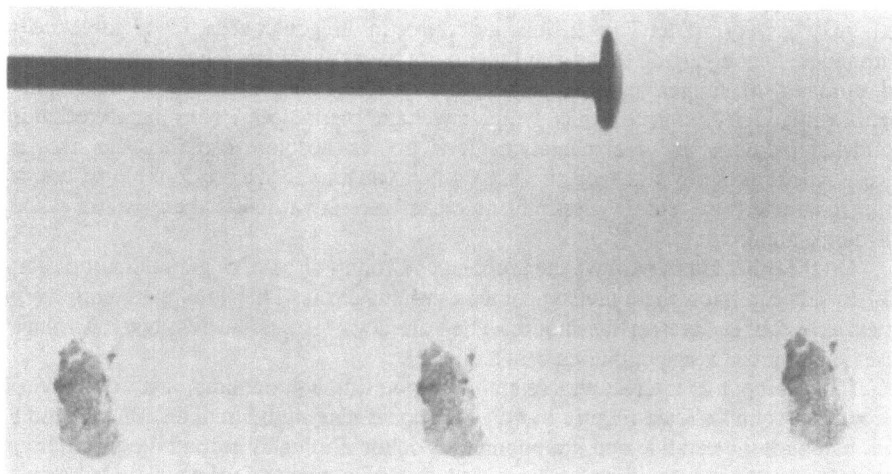

Figure 14-5 The minute size of a colonoscopic biopsy specimen is compared to that of an ordinary straight pin. × 6, HPS.

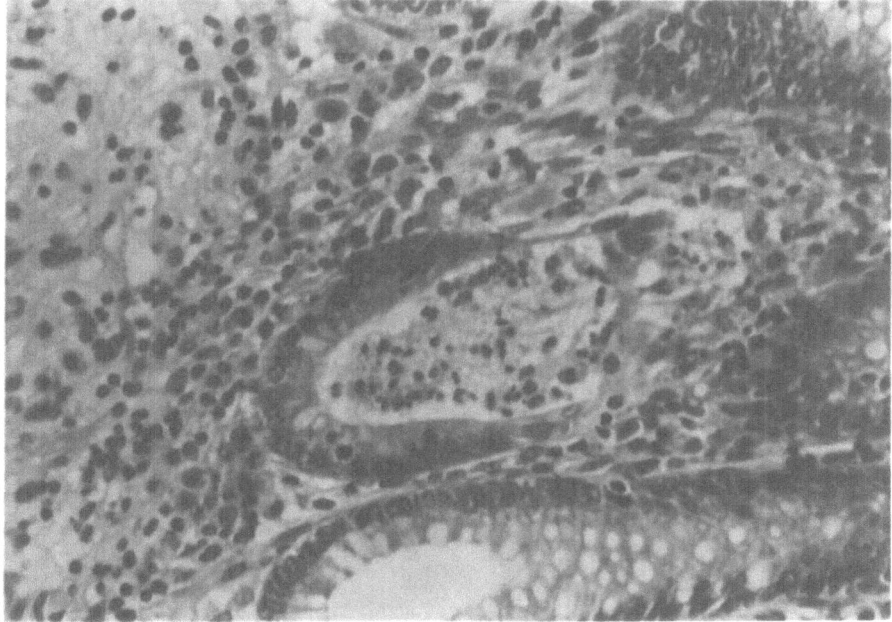

Figure 14-6 Ulcerative colitis biopsies sometimes include crypt abscesses, with neutrophils collected in the basal lumens. × 400, HPS.

granulation tissue with mucosa and it is not a hyperplastic proliferative or neoplastic reaction (Figure 14-7). Pseudopolyps are much more common in ulcerative colitis although they do occur in granulomatous colitis. Table 14-2 is a differential table of gross and microscopic changes found more in ulcerative or more in granulomatous colitis.

In the quiescent case, or in the case that has responded to therapy, the changes, if any, may be very subtle. They include a decrease in the goblet cells, fewer goblet cells with mucus in comparison to the cells that do not have any mucus. They include increased numbers of lamina propria leukocytes including all major types, statistically significantly increased neutrophils, lymphocytes and plasma cells. They include cellular epithelial pyknosis and fragmentation. It is not an absolute certainty that this is ulcerative colitis or any other specific entity unless you have seen a previous biopsy that is more characteristic. But in clinically quiescent ulcerative colitis there is still some histologic abnormality.

On the other hand, we have the problem of Crohn's disease, or granulomatous colitis. In this condition there are sometimes aphthous ulcers. They look apparently very much like canker sores in the mouth. They are always supposed to suggest Crohn's disease and it is a very popular current subject.

In the biopsy of the rectum or sigmoid, if you find a granuloma, it is very easy to recognize Crohn's disease (Figure 14-8). In the correlative studies that Dr Korelitz and I did, comparing ulcerative and granulomatous colitis using all histopathologic criteria, the only statistically significant feature that clearly indicated Crohn's disease beyond doubt was the granuloma in the lamina propria of the colon or rectum. There are some other less totally satisfying diagnostic findings. For example, notice the mucous goblet

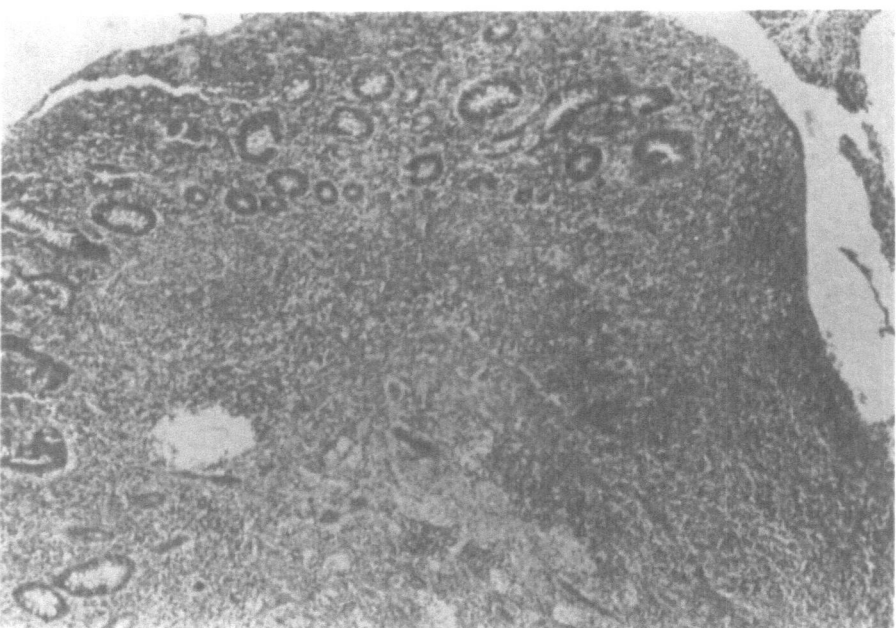

Figure 14-7 The rounded pseudopolyp is characteristically largely composed of inflamed granulation tissue. × 100, HPS.

Table 14-2
Gross and Microscopic Changes in Inflammatory Bowel Disease

	Ulcerative Colitis	Granulomatous Colitis
Gross Changes		
Ulcers	More numerous and extensive	May be absent
Cobblestone mucosa	Not usual	Present
Skip areas of inflammation	No	Yes
Pseudopolyps ulcers	More common	Less common
Aphthous ulcers	No	Yes
Anal and perineal fissures and fistulas	Less common	More common
Microscopic Changes		
Decreased mucosal goblet cells	Yes	Often no
Neutrophils overrun mucosa	Yes	No
Lymphangiectasia	No	Yes
Lymphoid nodules, in submucosa > mucosa	No	Yes
Crypt lesions	Abscess (PMNs)	Eos and macrophages
Muscularis propria involved	No	Yes
Knife-shaped fistulas	No	Yes
Cicatrization	No	Yes
Microscopic skip areas	No	Yes
Granulomas	No	Yes

cells are maintained in abundance. That happens in Crohn's disease, and is unlike what happens in ulcerative colitis. They decrease in ulcerative colitis.

Secondly, you have edema of the lamina propria separating the crypt base from the muscularis mucosae and you have lymphangiectasia. Also there are lymph nodules in Crohn's disease all through the gastrointestinal (GI) tract, both in the mucosa and submucosa. Sometimes there are more in the submucosa than the mucosa. That is Morson's criterion which indicates the likelihood of Crohn's disease.

If there are crypt lesions, they may be crypt abscesses with neutrophils. But with a polychrome or Giemsa stain, one might find a typical crypt lesion characteristic of Crohn's disease made up of eosinophilic leukocytes and macrophages. That is not seen in ulcerative colitis. One does not make a diagnosis by crypt abscess of either ulcerative or granulomatous colitis. It is an ornament to the diagnosis because crypt abscesses occur in heavy metal poisoning, in uremia, in pellagra, and a variety of other conditions.

Dr Korelitz and I have written about cell counts in ulcerative and granulomatous colitis. Leukocyte counts are important in the follow-up and in the distinction between quiescent ulcerative and granulomatous colitis, in clinical remission and sigmoidoscopically negative. If you do a cell count, the sigmoidoscopic biopsy will show a significantly increased number of neutrophils. It may be ulcerative colitis quiescent clinically, radiologically and endoscopically but there are more neutrophils in the lamina propria than there should be. In contrast, in Crohn's disease, in the uninvolved segment with negative sigmoidoscopy, the lamina propria has significantly increased macrophages or histiocytes (Table 14-3). It is as if histiocytes or macrophages had mobilized through the whole gastrointestinal tract, and only in places do they congregate and form a granuloma.

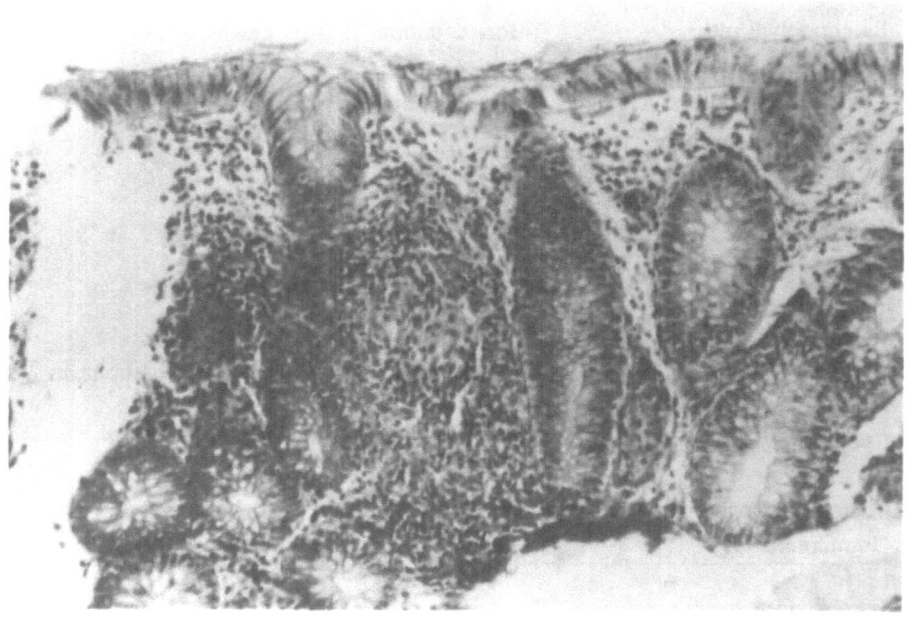

Figure 14-8 A rectal mucosal biopsy contains a typical granuloma of Crohn's disease. × 200, HPS.

Table 14-3
Statistically Significant Cell Count Differences Between Sigmoidoscopically Negative Cases of Ulcerative (UC) and Granulomatous Colitis (GC).

	UC		GC		Controls
Macrophages	8.5	<	10.5	>	7.8
Mast cells	0.39	>	0.27		
	0.39			>	0.1
Plasma cells	45.4	>	39.9	<	50.3
Eosinophils	0.04	>	0		
Neutrophils	3.2	>	0.86		

BIBLIOGRAPHY

Korelitz BI, Sommers SC: Rectal biopsy studies in Crohn's disease (histopathology and cell counts). In *The Management of Crohn's Disease*. Amsterdam, Excerpta Med, 1975, pp 13–17.

Korelitz BI, Sommers SC: Rectal biopsy in patients with Crohn's disease. *JAMA* 237:2742–2744, 1977.

Laufer I, Costopoulos L: Early lesions of Crohn's disease. *Am J Roentgenol* 130:307–311, 1978.

Sommers SC, Korelitz BI: Mucosal-cell counts in ulcerative and granulomatous colitis. *Am J Clin Pathol* 63:359–365, 1975.

Tucker PC, Webster PD, Kilpatrick FM: Amebic colitis mistaken for inflammatory bowel disease. *Arch Int Med* 135:681–685, 1975.

15 Where Has Colonoscopy Had Its Greatest Value in the Management of Inflammatory Bowel Disease?

Jerome D. Waye, MD

The greatest impact endoscopy has had in inflammatory bowel disease (IBD) is in the further definition of radiographically discovered abnormalities. The role of colonoscopy will be discussed in surveillance, but actually the greatest impact of endoscopy is in the elucidation of abnormalities on barium enema x-ray examination. Mass lesions seen on the x-ray may include:

1. Retained stool
2. Polyps and pseuodpolyps
3. Strictures
4. Cancer.

Stool is usually not considered to be a major problem in patients with IBD who have diarrhea. However, in the patient with chronic long-standing IBD to whom one does not wish to give a vigorous cathartic preparation, multiple small defects or irregularities on the wall of the colon caused by retained fecal material may occur.

Pseudopolyps appear as small, discrete, round sessile polyps on the x-ray and appear as a smooth small polyp on the colonoscopic examination. Multiple pseudopolyps, both sessile and pedunculated, are frequently present in the same colon. Pseudopolyps may appear in all shapes and varieties, and the endoscopist may have difficulty in making the correct diagnosis from viewing them directly. Some pseudopolyps may be quite large and almost occlude the narrowed lumen in patients with chronic IBD. Although the surface of pseudopolyps is usually smooth and glistening, this is not always so. Occasionally, large pseudopolyps may consist of reactive granulation tissue whose surface is irregular and quite friable. Upon direct visualization, such a lesion can appear remarkably similar in gross appearance to cancer of the colon. The only certain method of differentiating a large irregular pseudopolyp from cancer is by microscopic examination of tissue obtained by endoscopic biopsy. A tissue sample of any portion of a pseudopolyp will confirm the diagnosis, since the histopathologic differentiation is complete. The question frequently arises as to whether pseudopolyps occur more frequently in one type of IBD than in another. In reviewing our studies with IBD, we found that the incidence of pseudopolyps is substantial. About one-third of all patients with IBD have pseudopolyps, and they are equally distributed in patients with ulcerative and granulomatous colitis. Prior reports that pseudopolyps mean ulcerative colitis are not correct. Pseudopolyps do, therefore, occur in both diseases. When pseudopolyps are multiple and scattered, it is impossible to biopsy them all. Certain criteria may be used to decide which pseudopolyps should be biopsied. They include those which:

1. are over 1.0 cm in diameter
2. are friable or bleeding
3. appear grossly different in coloration from surrounding pseudopolyps
4. have an irregular surface.

The second radiographic abnormality that is frequently noted is a stricture in a patient with long-standing IBD. The axiom is that a stricture in a patient with ulcerative colitis is carcinoma until proven otherwise. In many instances, with the use of colonoscopy, we can prove otherwise and prevent the patient from having a total colonic resection. Narrowed segments of the colon lumen may be due to inflammation. The spasm associated with an active inflammation is usually distensible and may be easily intubated with the endoscope. Some strictures may be fibrotic because of previously healed inflammation, and carcinoma may present as a colon stricture in patients with chronic ulcerative colitis. X-ray evidence of a stricture may actually represent colon narrowing due to exuberant growth of pseudopolyps. Whenever strictures are encountered in patients with chronic ulcerative colitis, colonoscopy should be performed to permit visual inspection of the area and to collect material for cytology and histopathologic study. It is not sufficient only to visualize the distal-most portion of a stricture; the entire lumen must be seen, as well as the proximal edge. Without a complete and thorough endoscopic evaluation, a carcinoma that is mainly submucosal can be overlooked.

The endoscopist should not be complacent about the visual impression gained by direct inspection, for this may be misleading. It is essential that biopsies and/or cytology be performed. If strictures cannot be intubated with the standard-sized endoscope, a smaller (pediatric) instrument should be used. A judgment as to the benignity of a stricture cannot be properly made unless the entire stricture and its proximal margin are visualized, brushed, and/or biopsied. There is no need for operative resection of a stricture (usually associated with a total colectomy) if that stricture is adequately inspected and found to be benign. Occasionally, strictures and pseudopolyps are present simultaneously. This presents no greater problem in diagnosis than if the two existed separately. The same criteria must be used by the examining physician in assessing each stricture and pseudopolyp.

Strictures may also occur in granulomatous colitis with the same frequency as seen in ulcerative colitis. Approximately 10% of all patients with IBD will have localized segments of narrowing in the colon. Most strictures are benign and are either inflammatory or fibrotic. Carcinoma should be suspected if strictures are not typically benign on endoscopy. One may use brush cytology or pinch biopsies, but if the stricture is not typically benign to gross visual examination it should be highly suspect. Typical cancers in the noncolitic bowel usually have a typical appearance. Cancer in patients with long-standing ulcerative colitis usually have the same appearance as those occurring in the normal bowel—that is, the tumor is bulky and has surface irregularity and friability. However, early cancer may be flatter than the usual malignant tumor because these colitic cancers have a different genesis than those occurring in the noncolitic bowel. Because of this, one must suspect a stricture that cannot be intubated, that has an abrupt shelf-like margin, that is friable, or that has an abrupt caliber change.

The greatest impact of endoscopy in IBD, therefore, is in the evaluation of abnormalities demonstrated on the barium enema examination. This usually means the elucidation of radiographic filling defects or of strictures. An additional benefit of colonoscopy is in the preoperative evaluation of patients with Crohn's disease.* Knowledge of the total distal extent of disease enables the surgeon to plan his operative resection properly to include the total area of inflamed bowel, rather than to rely on the notoriously poor technique of disease-extent estimation from examining the serosal aspect of the bowel.

Colonoscopy may also be of great benefit in enabling the clinician to render a specific differential diagnosis when all other techniques have failed. At present there are many endoscopic criteria to assist in making the proper diagnosis in most patients with IBD. Mucosal granularity and friability are present in both types of IBD but occur more commonly in ulcerative colitis than in granulomatous colitis. The surface mucosa in ulcerative colitis is usually diffusely ulcerated, giving rise to the edematous surface called "granularity," as well as to spontaneous bleeding. However, the ulcerations are microscopic and only rarely may be appreciated grossly, even with the multifold magnification of colonoscopy. Ulcers in granulomatous colitis, on the other hand, are usually more discrete and larger, thus making them easier to see with the naked eye or flexible fiberoptic colonoscope. If the diseases were renamed today, we would give the name "ulcerative colitis" to Crohn's disease, since we see more actual ulcers in granulomatous colitis than are grossly visible on the mucosal surface. Very few patients with ulcerative colitis have skip areas, and none have cobblestoning of the mucosa.

The data concerning dysplasia in patients with chronic ulcerative colitis are confusing. Biopsies obtained from sigmoidoscopy and colonoscopy may be interpreted differently by various pathologists, since there is neither uniformity of opinion nor controls of histopathologic reading of dysplasia. In New York pathologists report less dysplasia than in England, but "blinded" studies have not been performed. The data concerning the relationship of dysplasia to cancer are striking and believable. However, the value of multiple endoscopic biopsies will depend on whether the pathologist over- or under-reads

---

*Editor's note: This is controversial.

the entity of dysplasia. The true value, number of biopsies, and the proper intervals for their performance are not known at the present time.

SUMMARY

The greatest impact of endoscopy in patients with IBD has been in the further evaluation of abnormalities demonstrated on a barium enema x-ray examination. Filling defects can be further identified and biopsied if desired; strictures can be visualized and completely characterized. Endoscopy may also assist in the differential diagnosis of granulomatous or ulcerative colitis, as well as in the delineation of the extent of disease in preoperative pâtients with Crohn's disease. The role of endoscopy in the surveillance of cancer is currently being scrutinized by several investigators to determine its role in the early detection of carcinoma in patients with chronic ulcerative colitis.

BIBLIOGRAPHY

Cook MG, Goligher JC: Carcinoma and epithelial dysplasia complicating ulcerative colitis. *Gastroenterology* 68:1127–1136, 1975.

Crowson TD, Ferrante WF, Gathright JB Jr: Colonoscopy: inefficacy for early carcinoma detection in patients with ulcerative colitis. *JAMA* 236:2651–2652, 1976.

Greenstein AJ, Sachar DB, Pucillo A, et al: Cancer in universal and left-sided ulcerative colitis: clinical and pathologic features. *Mt Sinai J Med* 46:25–32, 1979.

Hunt RH, Teague RH, Swarbrick ET, et al: Colonoscopy in the management of colonic strictures. *Br Med J* 11:360–361, 1975.

Waye JD: The role of colonoscopy in the differential diagnosis of inflammatory bowel disease. *Gastrointest Endosc* 23:150–154, 1977.

Waye JD: Colitis, cancer and colonoscopy. *Med Clin North Am* 62:211–224, 1978.

Waye JD: Endoscopy in inflammatory bowel disease. Clinics in gastroenterology (in press).

16 The Significance of Microgranulomas in Crohn's Disease

Heidi Z. Rotterdam, MD

This chapter is based on the examination of rectal biopsies in patients with Crohn's disease, all of whom had negative sigmoidoscopy. The diagnosis of Crohn's disease was based on x-ray findings and clinical presentation. Of 99 patients, 14 showed granulomatous lesions in grossly normal rectal mucosa. This incidence of 14% is higher than any reported previously. In previous reports 0% to 8% of biopsies showed granulomas in normal rectal mucosa. The difference between the results of others and ours is explained by differences of patient populations and differing criteria for what constitutes a granuloma. Of these 14 cases with granulomas in our series, more than half had very small granulomas, which were either missed at the initial reading or called "questionable granuloma." We call these microgranulomas and sometimes find them in association with the typical granuloma, sometimes without.

Before discussing the morphology of the microgranulomas, let us review the features of the usual mature granuloma. A well-developed mature granuloma is easily recognizable at low power (Figure 16-1). The mucosal surface is usually intact and the granuloma causes no bulging. Other features of Crohn's disease such as lymphangiectasia, lymphoid aggregates, and an increase of inflammatory cells are usually present. A mature granuloma is composed of large epithelioid histiocytes with abundant pink cytoplasm and also giant cells with multiple nuclei. Lymphocytes are interspersed but are located mainly at the periphery of the granuloma. Mature granulomas vary in size. Figure 16-2 shows a small granuloma in a rectal biopsy from another patient with grossly normal rectal mucosa at sigmoidoscopy. Although small, the granuloma is well defined and includes a giant cell. Lymphocytes and histiocytes are increased in number in the lamina propria. In spite of its small size, this granuloma is easily recognizable because it is compact, sharply demarcated from the surrounding inflammatory infiltrate, and composed of large histiocytes and only a few interspersed lymphocytes. A microgranuloma is not clearly visible under low power, but only under higher magnification. Returning to Figure 16-1, we also see a region of cryptal separation next to the mature granuloma and widening of the interstitium at the lower margin of the biopsy. Under high power a loose, poorly outlined aggregate of histiocytes, which are smaller than the ones in the mature granuloma can be seen (Figure 16-3). They are less epithelioid and are intermixed with mature lymphocytes.

Figure 16-4 shows a biopsy with a microgranuloma that appears only as a dense area. The remainder of the mucosa is pale because of edema. A poorly defined collection of histiocytes mixed with lymphocytes is seen under the surface epithelium, which is infiltrated by a few leukocytes.

How microscopic can a microgranuloma be? In Figure 16-5 it is composed of only about four histiocytes aggregated with a few lymphocytes. It lifts itself only poorly from the background, and it is a matter of perception and nomenclature as to what to call this lesion. Some refer to it as "focal lesion" or "histiocytic aggregate." We call it microgranuloma and so far have only seen it in Crohn's disease with typical radiologic and clinical findings.

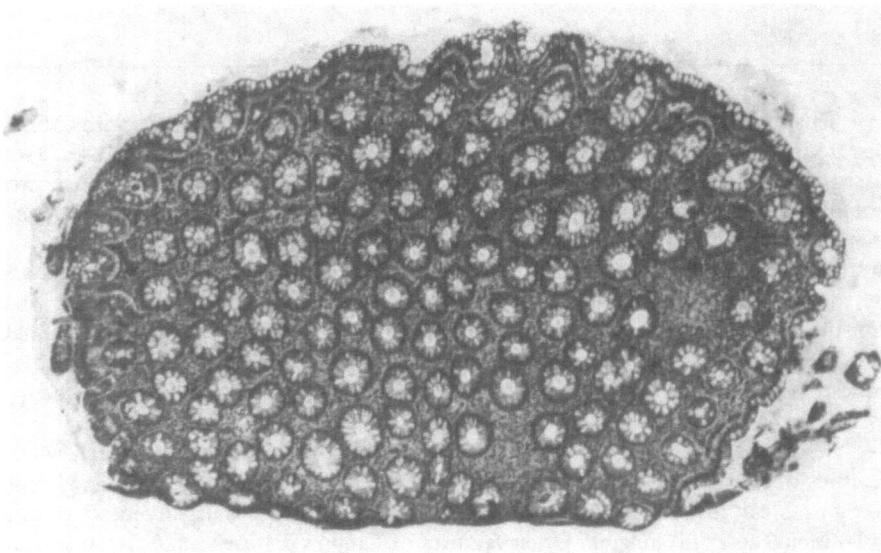

Figure 16-1 Rectal biopsy with mature granuloma on the right and a microgranuloma at the bottom.

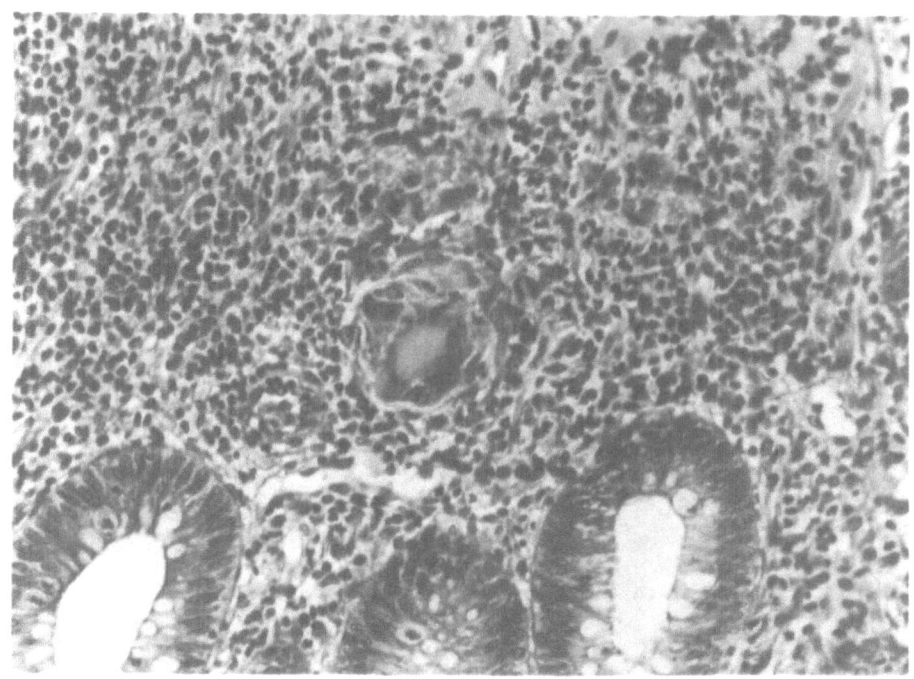

Figure 16-2 Rectal biopsy with small granuloma.

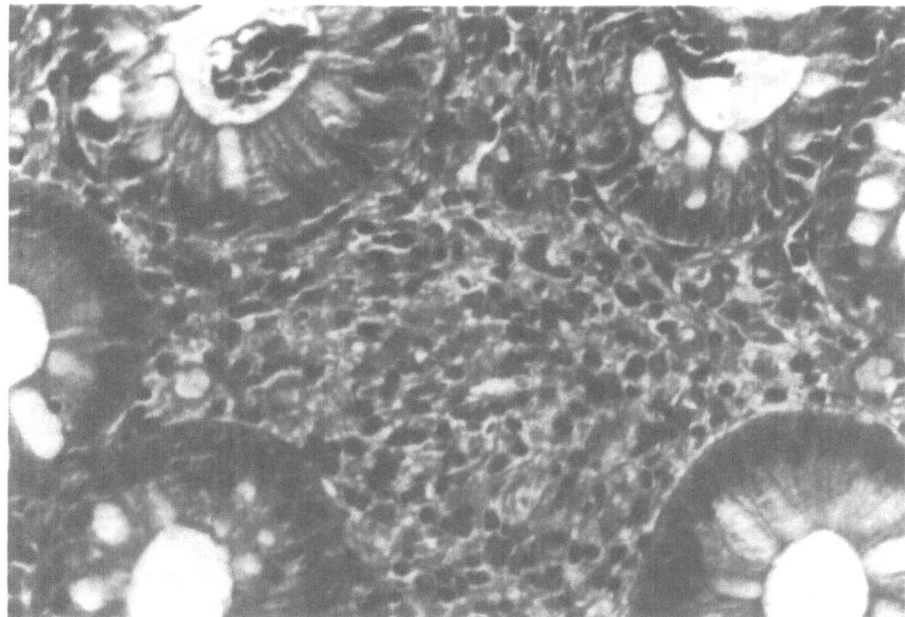

Figure 16-3 Rectal biopsy with microgranuloma.

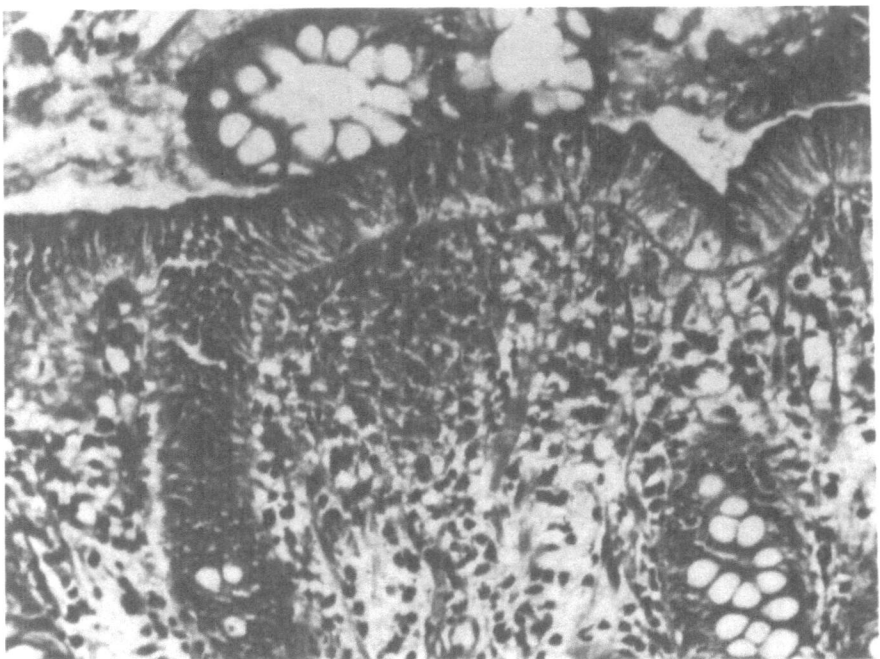

Figure 16-4   Rectal biopsy with microgranuloma under the surface epithelium.

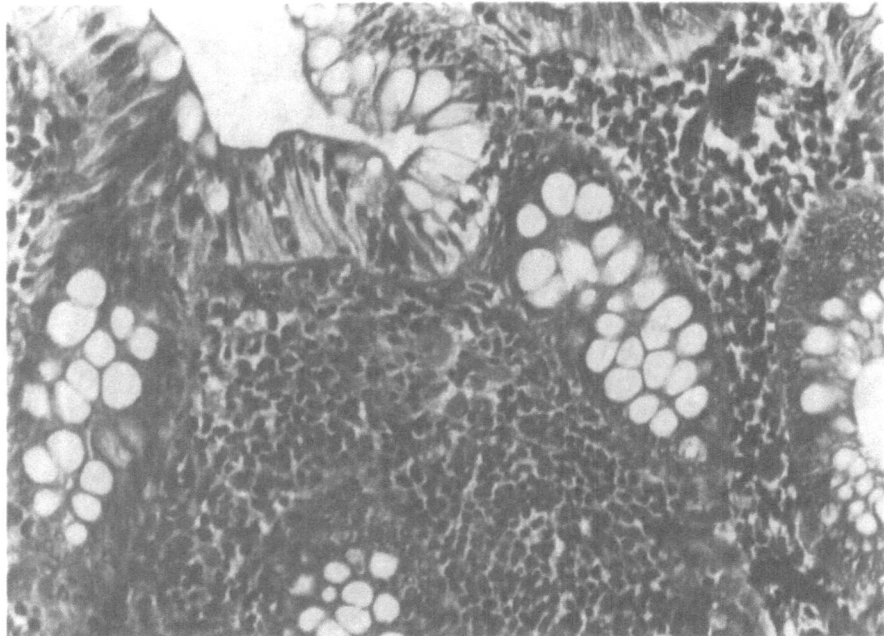

Figure 16-5   Rectal biopsy with microgranuloma under the surface epithelium.

In our experience most microgranulomas were located under the surface epithelium. A few were found in deeper regions of the mucosa. Microgranulomas should not be confused with tangentially-cut crypts or lymphoid aggregates with a germinal center. If in doubt, serial sections will help.

The concept of the microgranuloma is not new. Mallory's *Textbook of Pathology* in 1914 described the early lesion of tuberculosis as "early granuloma," in which histiocytes are smaller and less epithelioid than in a mature granuloma (Figure 16-6). There are no giant cells. The microgranuloma is a variant or probably a precursor of the granuloma. Whether every microgranuloma ultimately becomes a granuloma or whether it can regress, we do not know. To realize its existence increases our awareness and the number of positive diagnoses in rectal biopsies.

To summarize, microgranulomas have a loose composition, while mature granulomas are compact and sarcoid-like. Biopsies have to be examined under higher power and in multiple serial sections. We examine an average of 12 sections. Certainly, if we examined 100 sections of each biopsy, our yield would be still greater than it is at the present time. Microgranulomas are small, about 0.2 mm in diameter, while the granulomas are larger. Microgranulomas are most frequently found under the surface epithelium, while granulomas are generally found in deeper regions of the mucosa or submucosa. We have never found a microgranuloma in the submucosa, although most biopsies include a small portion of submucosal tissue. Microgranulomas are ill-defined

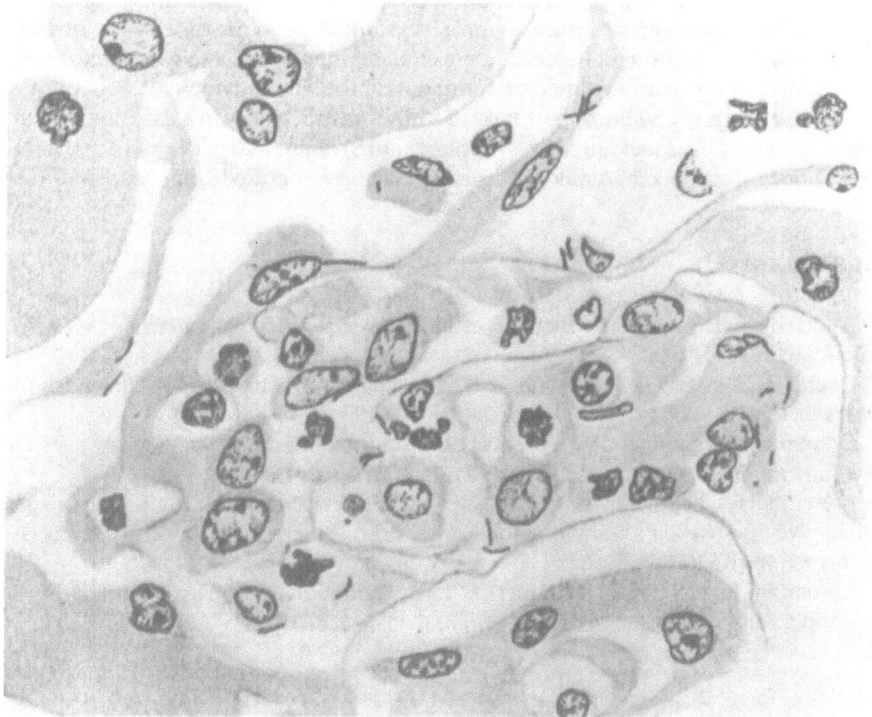

Figure 16-6 "Early granuloma" of tuberculosis (Mallory's *Textbook of Pathology* 1914).

because they have a fair number of lymphocytes mixed with histiocytes. Since lymphocytes are also diffusely scattered in the surrounding mucosa, the outline of microgranulomas appears blurred. The ratio of histiocytes to lymphocytes within the smallest lesion is only 2:1. In the granuloma, the predominant cell is the large histiocyte and only a few lymphocytes are interspersed. We found giant cells only in granulomas.

I mentioned the superficial location of the microgranuloma and would like to discuss its possible meaning in the light of what we know about the normal structure of the colonic crypt. The lower third of the crypt comprises the germinative zone in which cells are still undifferentiated. The goblet cell matures first. The resorptive cell, however, matures only toward the upper part of the crypt and is most frequent on the surface of the colonic mucosa. Whatever substance is resorbed from the lumen will first appear in the upper portion of the lamina propria. Thus it seems likely that the small microgranulomas located in this area develop in response to a factor that is resorbed through the surface epithelium.

One other feature that deserves comment is the possible association with lymphatics. In the small intestine, granulomas often develop in the wall of lymphatics. In the colon, lymphatics are intimately connected with the muscularis mucosae, but none reach upward into the mucosa. This is in contrast to the small intestine, where lymphatics are seen immediately under the surface. In the rectum, microgranulomas cannot possibly develop in the wall of the lymphatics, because there are no lymphatics in the upper two-thirds of the mucosa. The proximity of microgranulomas and surface epithelium of the colon on one hand, and of granulomas and lymphatics in the small intestine on the other hand, are not contradictory observations. A substance absorbed by the surface epithelium may evoke a granulomatous response under the surface, and its concentration in the lymph could result in granuloma formation in the wall of lymphatics.

We have recently had the opportunity to study a gastric biopsy in a patient who had Crohn's disease of the small intestine. We found microgranulomas in the gastric mucosa as well. Sometimes a microgranuloma develops around a ruptured crypt abscess.

BIBLIOGRAPHY

Anderson FH, Bogach A: Biopsies of large bowel in regional enteritis. *Can Med Assoc J* 98:150–153, 1968.

Dyer NH, Stansfeld AG, Dawson AM: The value of rectal biopsy in the diagnosis of Crohn's disease. *Scand J Gastroenterol* 5:491–496, 1970.

Goodman MJ, Skinner JM, Truelove SC: Abnormalities in the apparently normal bowel mucosa in Crohn's disease. *Lancet* 1:275–278, 1976.

Present DH, Chapman ML, Cohen N, et al: The correlation of sigmoidoscopy and rectal valve biopsy in granulomatous disease of the small bowel (abstract). *Gastroenterology* 52:1113, 1967.

Rotterdam H, Korelitz BI, Sommers SC: Microgranulomas in grossly normal rectal mucosa in Crohn's disease. *Am J Clin Pathol* 67:550–554, 1977.

17 Scanning Electronmicroscopic Appearance of "Early" Lesions in Crohn's Disease

Robert R. Rickert, MD

The pathologic features of inflammatory bowel disease (IBD) and the differential features which distinguish them have been well documented.[1,2,3] The pathologist usually sees Crohn's disease in an advanced state of morphologic evolution. In this chapter attention will be focused on what perhaps has naively been designated as the "early" lesion of Crohn's disease. There is no evidence documenting that the findings to be described are truly "early." What will be discussed are "small" lesions of Crohn's disease; small but in many instances at least recognizable macroscopically.

The recognition of these minute ulcerative lesions in Crohn's disease is by no means new. As early as 1953, Brooke[4] described these in resected surgical specimens and called them aphthoid ulcers because of their gross similarity to the oral lesions seen in aphthous stomatitis. They are regarded by some as the earliest grossly recognizable lesions of Crohn's disease,[5] and vary from barely visible up to 3 mm in diameter. Since some of the smallest lesions cannot be recognized grossly, perhaps they should be designated as the minute or microulcerative lesion of Crohn's disease rather than the aphthoid ulcer. They usually appear grossly as tiny red mucosal spots which sometimes appear to be simply surgical artifacts or petechiae due to handling of the bowel. But if one examines the center, one can often see a small white collection of material on the ulcerated surface which turns out to be a minute streamer of mucopurulent exudate (Figure 17-1). Sometimes these seem to surmount a small nodule of edematous submucosa, but often they are seen in the background of grossly normal mucosa.

Histologically this lesion also has a very characteristic appearance (Figure 17-2). It is a small focus of ulceration with a "streamer" of mucopurulent material at the base. One of the interesting features of these leions is that they are commonly located over a lymphoid aggregate. Sometimes it appears to be a previously present but hyperplastic lymphoid follicle. In some of these lymphoid aggregates, we have been able to identify granulomas, both of the fully developed type and also the so-called microgranuloma. Another characteristic histologic feature of the lesion is the epithelium at either side of the defect which appears to be hyperplastic and regenerative, as if in an effort to heal. Actually, in examining some of these minute red spots microscopically and serially sectioning them, we found that apparently the lesions can heal.

Because of our interest in IBD, we have seen these small "aphthoid" ulcers for a long time. We thought it would be valuable and interesting to study the frequency, distribution, and morphology of these lesions.[6] In a period of about a year and a half, we had an opportunity to study 18 surgical specimens from 17 patients ranging in age from 16 to 75 years. Of these 18 specimens, 12 were from patients for whom this was the initial surgical procedure. Ten of these specimens were portions of the terminal ileum and right colon, and two were total proctocolectomy specimens. In six patients the surgical treatment was for recurrent disease. Three of these were portions of small bowel and three were contiguous segments of small and large bowel.

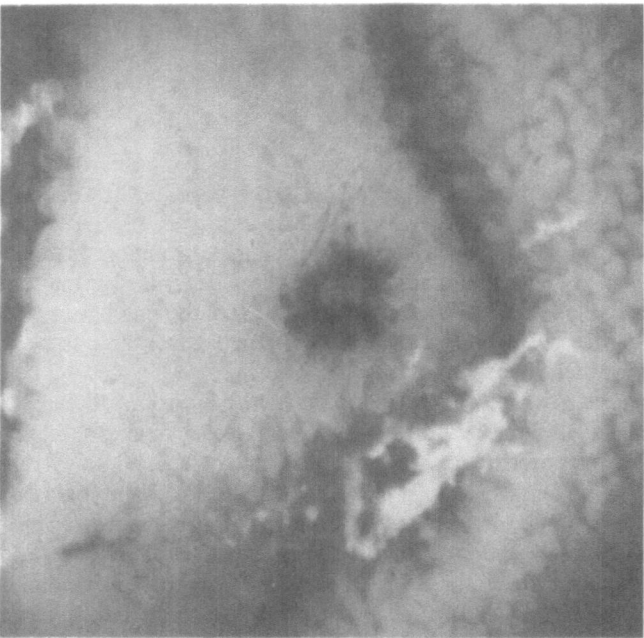

Figure 17-1   Ulcer of ileum seen with dissecting microscope. Ulcer measures 0.25 mm and is surrounded by cuff of congested mucosa.

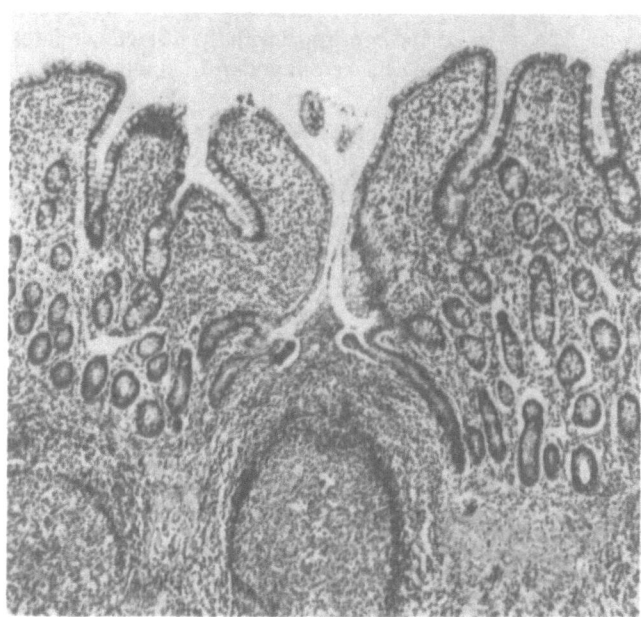

Figure 17-2A Lightmicroscopic view of ileal ulcer. Note underlying hyperplastic lymphoid nodule.

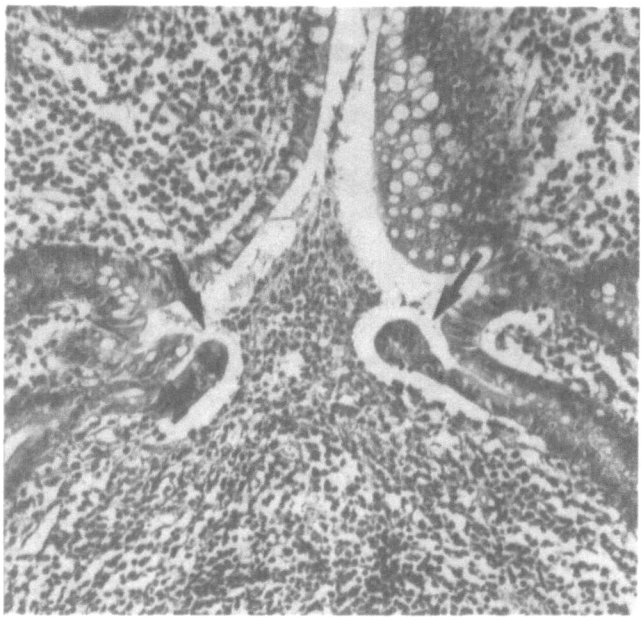

Figure 17-2B Higher power of Figure 17-2A. Note inflammatory "streamer" overlying ulcer base and regenerating epithelium at ulcer margins (arrows).

The specimens were initially examined with a hand lens. Lesions suspected of being minute ulcers were then reviewed and confirmed with the dissecting microscope. Of the 18 specimens, characteristic microulcers were found in 14 in mucosa which grossly was either normal or only focally edematous. In two of the specimens we found lesions only in grossly diseased mucosa, and in only two specimens were there no microulcers. These small lesions were more easily recognized in ideal than colonic mucosa, although in both of our proctocolectomy specimens we were able to recognize ulcers. The number of lesions varied from two to three to as many as 20 to 30.

Having gained some understanding of the fully developed lesion from our gross and light microscopic studies, we elected to study them with the scanning electronmicroscope. The scanning electronmicroscope proved especially valuable in the study because of the ability to detect surface phenomena at high magnification and with excellent resolution. The scanning electronmicroscope provides an excellent view of these microulcers (Figure 17-3). In the ileum the ulcer appears as a small mucosal defect with the surrounding villi arranged in a petal-like configuration. In the central pit, granular material is noted, which represents the inflammatory "streamer." Most of the villi at a distance from the ulcer appear quite normal but those immediately surrounding the ulcer may exhibit some rather unusual changes. The lesions are similar when seen in the colon (Figure 17-4). However, they are not as structurally interesting because the surrounding mucosa is much less complex and does not undergo the same type of changes.

Although we initially chose the scanning electronmicroscope as a medium for studying the ulcers themselves, we soon learned that additional information was available in the adjacent mucosa. We noted a variety of villous abnormalities, including blunting and

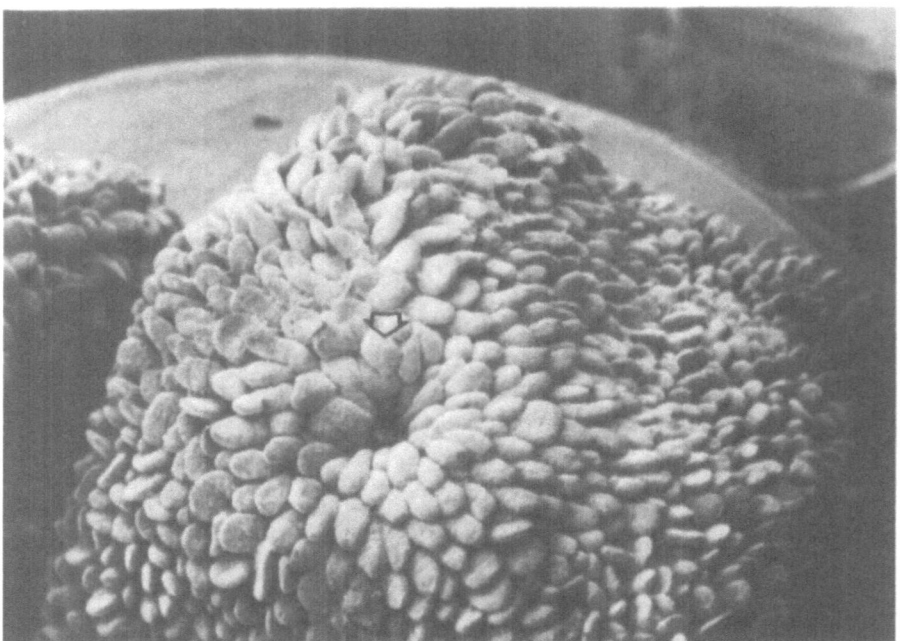

Figure 17-3A Ileal ulcer (0.2 mm) seen with scanning electronmicroscope. Note petal-like arrangement of surrounding villi. Villi at 12 o'clock (arrow) are blunted and fused.

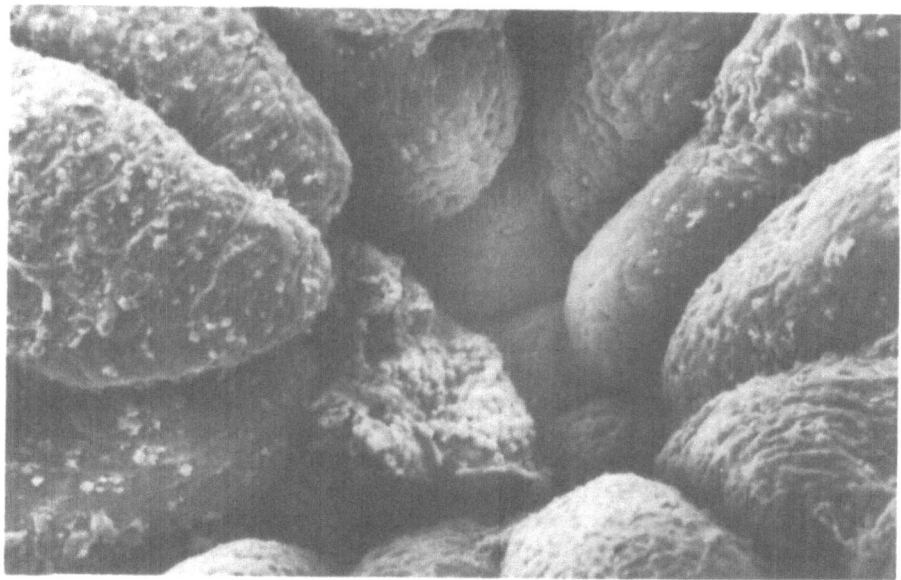

Figure 17-3B Higher magnification of ulcer in Figure 17-3A. Nodule of granular material in center corresponds to inflammatory "streamer" seen with light microscope (Figure 17-2B).

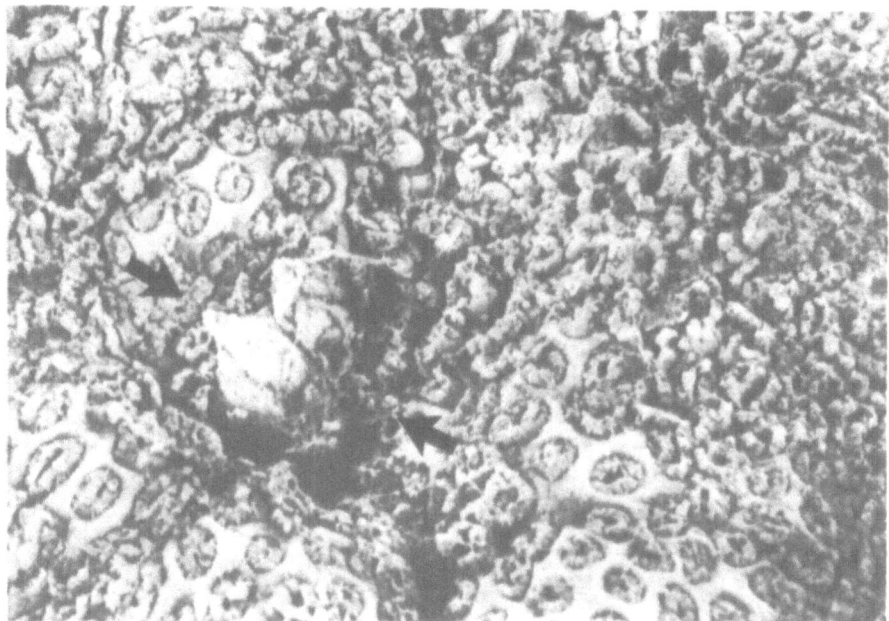

Figure 17-4 Colonic ulcer (0.2 mm) seen with scanning electronmicroscope (arrows). Adjacent mucosa is apparently normal.

fusion (Figure 17-5). This surrounding cuff of alteration varied from a single row of distorted villi to a more diffuse change. The extent of the villous abnormality tended to increase with increasing size of the ulcer. In addition to blunting and fusion, there were occasional examples of actual intervillous cellular bridging. This observation was subsequently confirmed in a review of the light microscopic material. Of interest was the fact that this cellular bridging may occur not only adjacent to the microulcerative lesion but also occasionally in mucosa not related to an ulcer. This may represent a nonspecific repair response to mucosal injury. The changes were not seen in control mucosa from terminal ileum which was taken from hemicolectomy specimens removed for carcinoma of the right colon.

The smallest ulcerative lesions we have seen have been less than the diameter of a single intestinal villus. Even at this extremely small size, the adjacent villi had already begun to fuse on the basis of cells crossing from one villus to the other.

The most important question concerning these observations is: What does this all mean? To begin with, the microulcerative lesions in Crohn's disease all seem to have the same appearance. They are highly characteristic, particularly with respect to their relationship to the underlying lymphoid tissue. Whether this is a lymphoid response to the lesion or whether it is ulceration of a preexisting lymphoid nodule undergoing hyperplastic change in a response to injury, is not known. It is very tempting to speculate, when looking at the activity within this lymphoid tissue, especially with the occasional presence of granulomas, that these foci represent the sites of antigen processing. Unfortunately we do not know whether the changes in the lymphoid tissue antedate or follow

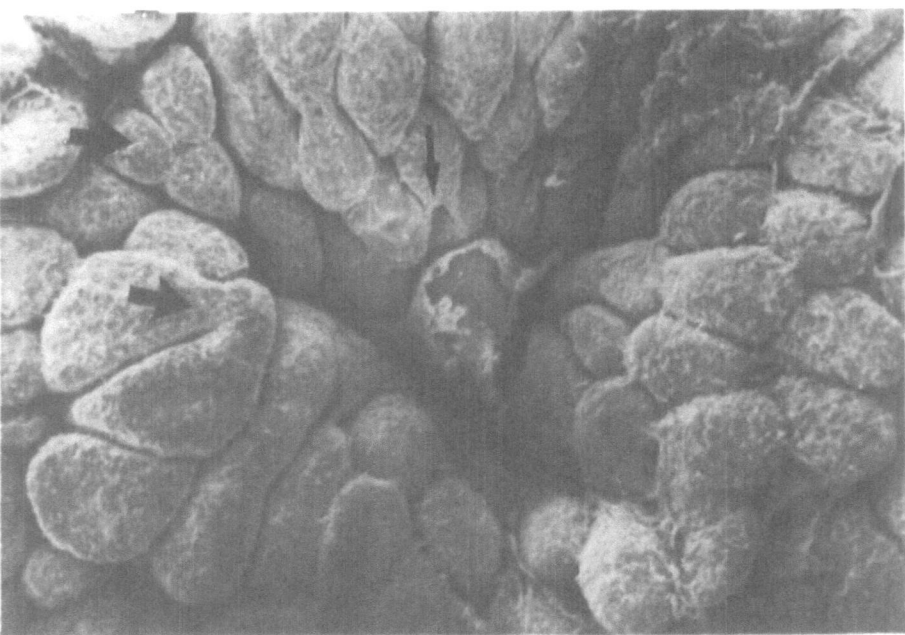

Figure 17-5A   Ileal ulcer (0.2 mm) seen with scanning electronmicroscope. Note central ulcer and surrounding villous changes including fusion (large arrows) and bridging (small arrow).

the ulcer formation. Nevertheless, it is interesting to speculate about the possible relationship of these minute lesions to the etiology and pathogenesis of Crohn's disease. If, as some have suggested, a transmissible agent is the cause of this disease, these foci must be considered as possible sites of the body's initial reaction to such an agent, or perhaps even the focus of entry.[7,8]

It has been documented that proven infectious diseases of the intestinal tract select lymphoid tissue as the site of major reaction. Typhoid fever is one example, another one is *Yersinia* infection. We have recently had an opportunity to study a case of acute *Yersinia* enteritis in which there were very similar microulcerative lesions overlying lymphoid follicles. We were able, with the transmission electronmicroscope, to identify the organisms at the base of the ulcer in the lymphoid tissue. Subsequent culture and serological tests proved the presence of *Yersinia*.[9] We are presently exploring this observation with Crohn's disease cases and are subserially studying several of these minute ulcerative lesions with the transmission electronmicroscope.

Another interesting area for consideration concerns the evolution of the lesion. There is little doubt that they sometimes heal, and there is also evidence from studying progressively larger and more typical ulcers of Crohn's disease. Lesions 2 mm to 3 mm in diameter have frequently been recognized grossly and more recently have been described radiographically.[10] It is these "larger" microulcers which perhaps deserve the designation of "aphthoid."

An important observation is the occurrence of these lesions in otherwise normal-appearing mucosa, often proximal to the major site of disease. It is likely that these lesions are more common and probably more widespread than suspected. Many are

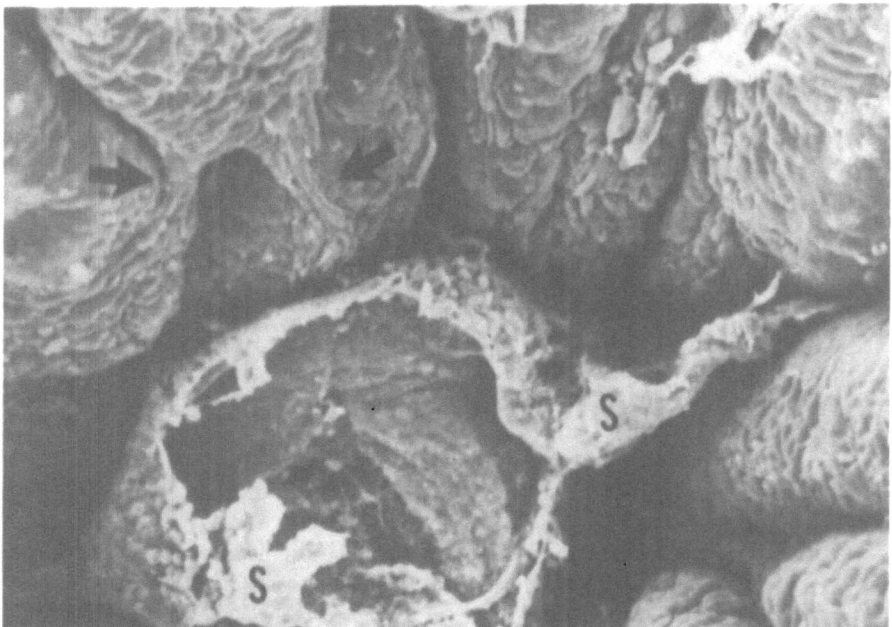

Figure 17-5B   High magnification of Figure 17-5A. Note intervillous bridging (arrows) and central ulcer with "streamer" (S).

probably present but undetected at the time of the original diagnosis. These may provide the morphologic source for clinical recurrence, in a sense representing the "seeds" for later recurrence. What we regard clinically as recurrent disease may actually represent maturation of lesions already present.

What we hope to have accomplished with this morphologic study is to point out some very focal features of the disease upon which to concentrate with more sophisticated techniques. Investigation is now being directed at immunologically characterizing the lymphoid tissue at the base of the ulcers. Because we know very little about the development and evolution of the morphologic changes in Crohn's disease, it would be preferable at this time to regard this ulcerative lesion as "small" rather than "early." We have continued this study to include additional cases, and these observations confirm and supplement our initial findings.[11]

SUMMARY

The pathology of advanced Crohn's disease (regional enteritis) has been studied in detail. The gross and microscopic features distinguishing it from ulcerative colitis and other inflammatory bowel diseases have been defined. Several very characteristic patterns of ulceration occur in Crohn's disease. One of these, which has received little attention in the literature, is believed by some to be the earliest macroscopic lesion of Crohn's disease. These distinctive lesions grossly resemble the aphthous ulcers frequently seen in the oral mucosa and, therefore, have been designated "aphthoid" ulcers. We have utilized the scanning electronmicroscope to study these early ulcerative lesions because this medium permits appreciation of their three-dimensional surface configuration.

In addition to providing an excellent technique to view these minute ulcers, the scanning electronmicroscope added morphologic details which were unsuspected. The findings were villous fusion caused by bridging by cells shown to be epithelial by lightmicroscopy, and an orderly, circular, petal-like arrangement of villi around the ulcers. The possible significance of these lesions in the pathogenesis of Crohn's disease has been discussed.

REFERENCES

1. Morson BC: Pathology of Crohn's disease. *Clin Gastroenterol* 1:265-277, 1972.

2. Lockhart-Mummary HE, Morson BC: Crohn's disease (regional enteritis) of the large intestine and its distinction from ulcerative colitis. *Gut* 1:87-105, 1960.

3. Hawk WA, Turnbull RB Jr, Farmer RG: Regional enteritis of the colon. *JAMA* 201:112.120, 1967.

4. Brooke BW: What is ulcerative colitis? *Lancet* 1:1220-1225, 1953.

5. Morson BC: The early histological lesion of Crohn's disease. *Proc R Soc Med* 65:71-72, 1972.

6. Rickert RR, Carter HW: The gross, light microscopic and scanning electron microscopic appearance of the early lesions of Crohn's disease. *Scan Electron Microsc* 2:179-186, 1977.

7. Mitchell DN, Rees RHW: Agent transmissible from Crohn's disease tissue. *Lancet* 2:168-171, 1970.

8. Mitchell DN, Rees RHW: Further observations on the transmissibility of Crohn's disease. *Ann NY Acad Sci* 278:546–559, 1976.

9. Douglass LE, Rickert RR, Carter HW: Light and electron microscopic studies of *Yersinia* enterocolitis. (In preparation.)

10. Laufer I, Costopoulos L: Early lesions of Crohn's disease. *Am J Roentgenol* 130:307–311, 1978.

11. Rickert RR, Carter HW: The "early" ulcerative lesions of Crohn's disease: correlative light and scanning electron microscopic studies. *J Clin Gastroenterol* 2:11–19, 1980.

18 Has There Been Any Progress in the X-ray Diagnosis and Differential Diagnosis of Inflammatory Bowel Disease?

Mansho T. Khilnani, MD

In the past few years dramatic developments have occurred in the science of radiology, particularly in the technological fields. Computerized tomography and ultrasonography have been influencing the course of medical diagnosis in many areas.

They have, however, been of limited value in the diagnosis of inflammatory bowel disease (IBD). Sometimes, it is possible to see the thick wall of the inflamed bowel. A similar appearance, however, can be produced by metastatic disease and lymphoma.

These two modalities have been of considerable help in differentiating inflammatory from neoplastic processes of the small bowel. The presence of marked lymphadenopathy in a patient with an inflammatory process, either of the small bowel or the colon, suggests that either the diagnosis of IBD is inaccurate, or that there is in addition, or as a complication, neoplasm associated with the IBD. It is also possible to differentiate retractile mesenteritis from IBD, especially Crohn's disease by computerized tomography. Increased thickness of the bowel wall favor Crohn's disease, while thickening of the mesentery and the deposition of a considerable amount of mesenteric fat favors the diagnosis of retractile mesenteritis.

Computerized tomography and ultrasonography have also been of help in the clinical management of these patients by providing a method of localization of abscesses for diagnosis as well as for percutaneous puncture. Ultrasonography can be useful in evaluating the liver parenchyma for the changes of cirrhosis.

A recent innovation of greater impact in the investigation of IBD has been the extensive use of double-contrast study with or without glucagon hypotonia. Other hypotonic drugs, such as atropine and propantheline, have been completely discarded because of associated undesirable side effects. This examination involves the use of high density barium, along with gas-forming effervescent granules or pills, for the investigation of the stomach and duodenum. For the colon study, high density adherent barium can be introduced with air almost simultaneously, to obtain a double-contrast barium enema. Glucagon, 0.01 to 0.5 mg, IV may be given for the stomach study, and 1.0 mg may be given IV for the colon study. Apart from one case of erythema multiforme and a few case reports of hypotension, no serious complications have been reported with the use of glucagon. There are no true contraindications to its use. Anaphylaxis has not been recorded to date with the use of this polypeptide.

Double contrast study, even though it has been used for a few decades, especially for the colon, has created a great deal of controversy among radiologists. Many radiology departments use it exclusively in investigating the digestive tract. Others show a greater or lesser degree of reservation and prefer to use the double-contrast method either in selected groups of patients or initially, followed by low-density barium study. It has in no way improved our ability to make a diagnosis of IBD where the older method failed to make a similar diagnosis. It has been the experience of many workers that the older method provided some information which is lost by the double-contrast study, especially if hypotonia has been induced.

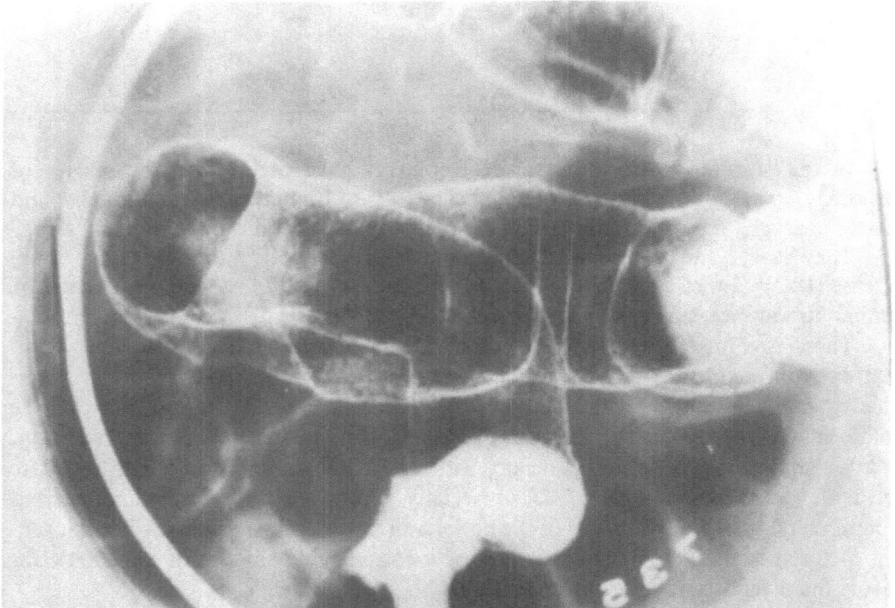

Figure 18-1 Idiopathic ulcerative colitis: Classical granular appearance of colon mucosa. The colon is shortened and narrowed.

Double-contrast study of the colon was initially suggested by workers in Sweden. The use of high-density, more adherent barium was popularized by Japanese radiologists for study of the stomach. Double-contrast study, as subsequently developed by investigators in this country, has made it possible to demonstrate certain subtle changes, not easily seen on the earlier two-stage barium enema and nonadherent barium meal study.

The double-contrast study of the colon has enabled us to show the minute, discrete aphthoid ulcers of early Crohn's disease and the diffuse ulceration presenting as granularity of the mucosa in idiopathic ulcerative colitis (Figure 18-1). Unfortunately, these findings are not pathognomonic of these conditions. As the aphthoid ulcers are more frequently seen in Crohn's disease and not in ulcerative colitis, the double-contrast study has helped in making this differential diagnosis with a greater degree of ease than previously (Figure 18-2). However, ulcers roentgenologically indistinguishable from these aphthoid ulcers may be seen in other types of colitis. Another very important differential point is that ulcerative colitis tends to be a continuous process extending cephalad from the rectum, while granulomatous colitis or Crohn's disease is often segmental and patchy in distribution in the involved segment (Figure 18-3). There are, however, a small number of cases where the presurgical differential between ulcerative colitis and granulomatous colitis cannot be made.

The double-contrast study also demonstrates finer detail of the normal colonic mucosa, such as the areae colonica, a mucosal folding produced by contractions of the muscularis mucosae. This is a transitory phenomenon. It has also been possible to demonstrate epithelial dysplasia, considered a precancerous condition, by the double-contrast technique, and differentiate spastic narrowing from a true organic stricture by the use of a hypotonic agent such as glucagon.

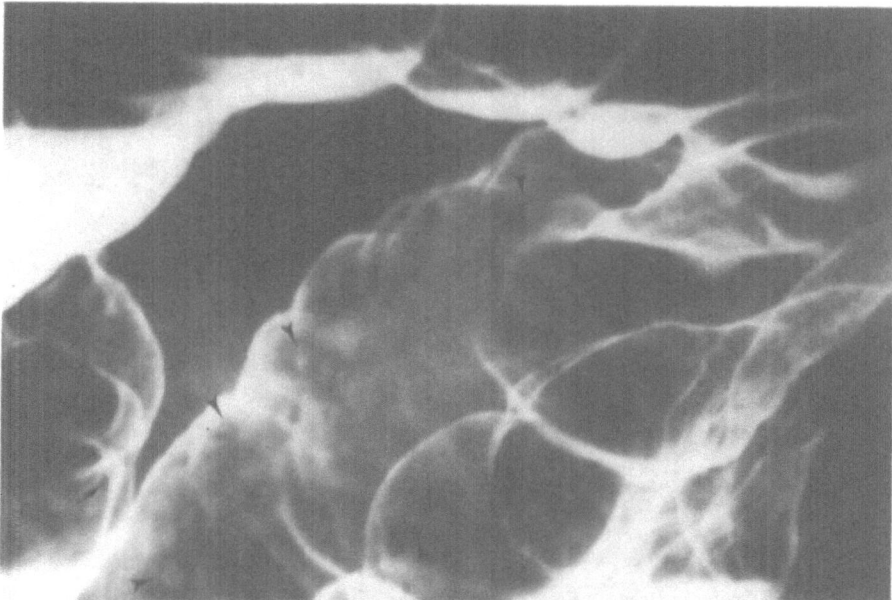

Figure 18-2 Crohn's disease: Many aphthous ulcers (minute ulcers surrounded by edema halo) are seen throughout this segment of the colon (arrow heads).

A not infrequent finding with a double-contrast enema are small nodular defects, especially in the right colon. These have been described as lymphoid nodules and, on biopsy, have proved to be lymphoid follicles. The significance of these nodular defects is not quite established. There is a feeling among some investigators that these may represent an early phase of Crohn's disease. However, these nodules may disappear spontaneously. These lymphoid nodules may actually represent a nonspecific response to any insult to the colon and should not be accepted as an early change of Crohn's disease. Pseudopolyps, mucosal bridging, and linear and serpiginous ulcers have been easier to demonstrate by the double-contrast enema.

In the stomach, double-contrast studies demonstrate minute ulcers, not obvious by older methods. The aphthoid ulcers of erosive gastritis may be clearly shown (Figure 18-4A & B). Similar aphthoid ulcers are also seen with Crohn's gastroduodenitis (Figure 18-5). The two types of ulcers and the two conditions are difficult to differentiate without clinical correlation and study of the small and large bowel. Double-contrast study of the upper gastrointestinal tract has shown that the estimated incidence of Crohn's disease of the stomach and duodenum, previously thought to be 4%, is probably five to eight times more frequent.

Another advantage of double-contrast study has been the reproducibility of the roentgen findings in the same patient at two different times.

Recently, there has been a renewed interest in the old technique of enteroclysis. In the past, a Cantor tube was introduced the night before and barium introduced when the tip of the catheter reached the point of interest. In the new technique, a tube is passed beyond the ligament of Treitz and 200 ml to 400 ml of barium mixture is introduced slowly. This is followed by injection of water, air, or methylcellulose. Water has the

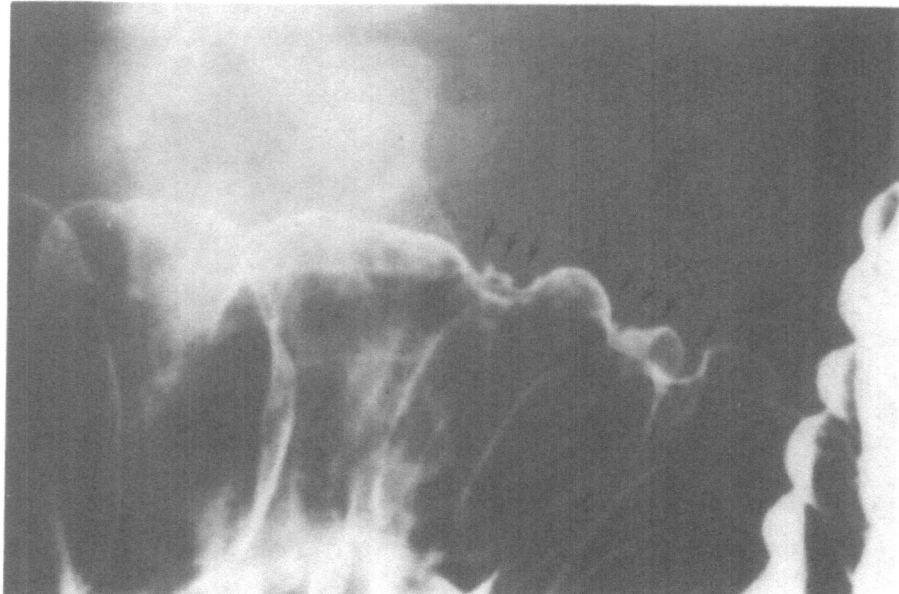

Figure 18-3 Crohn's disease: Focal involvement of the superior aspect of transverse colon (arrows). This would not have been as elegantly demonstrated by the older single-contrast barium study of the colon.

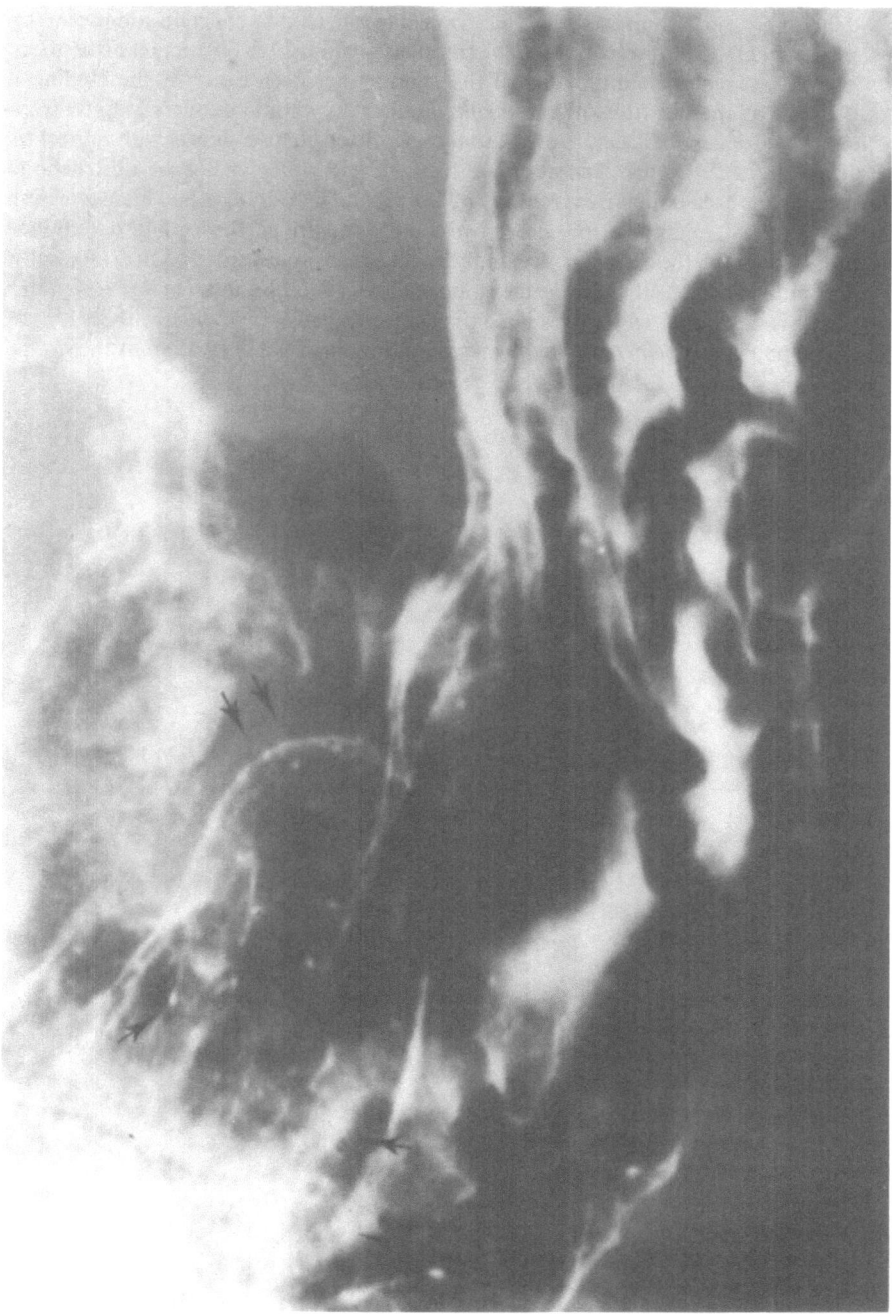

Figure 18-4 Erosive gastritis – two cases. Small bowel and colon were normal in both cases. A Multiple punctate ulcerations are seen on distorted, edematous mucosal folds of the antrum of the stomach (arrows). Confirmed on endoscopy.

112

disadvantage of diluting the barium in the small bowel, while the air may not be present at the site where the barium is present. Methylcellulose in a 0.5% concentration seems to be the best agent. The examination can be completed within 20 to 30 minutes after injection of contrast material. Intubation of the jejunum has been easier by the Herlinger modification of the old Bilbao-Dotter tube used for hypotonic duodenography. This method provides a more accurate evaluation of short segments of bowel with respect to the diagnosis of IBD, demonstration of fistulae, and other causes of obstruction. Enteroclysis has been popularized recently by Sellink and by Herlinger and his associates.

The surgical treatment for ulcerative colitis used to be the standard terminal ileostomy. Recently, the continent ileostomy has been the procedure of choice, especially in young individuals. As there are some complications with the continent ileostomy, the radiologist is now required to investigate the continent ileostomy pouch with its nipple valve. The pouch can be investigated by retrograde method via intubation of the stoma

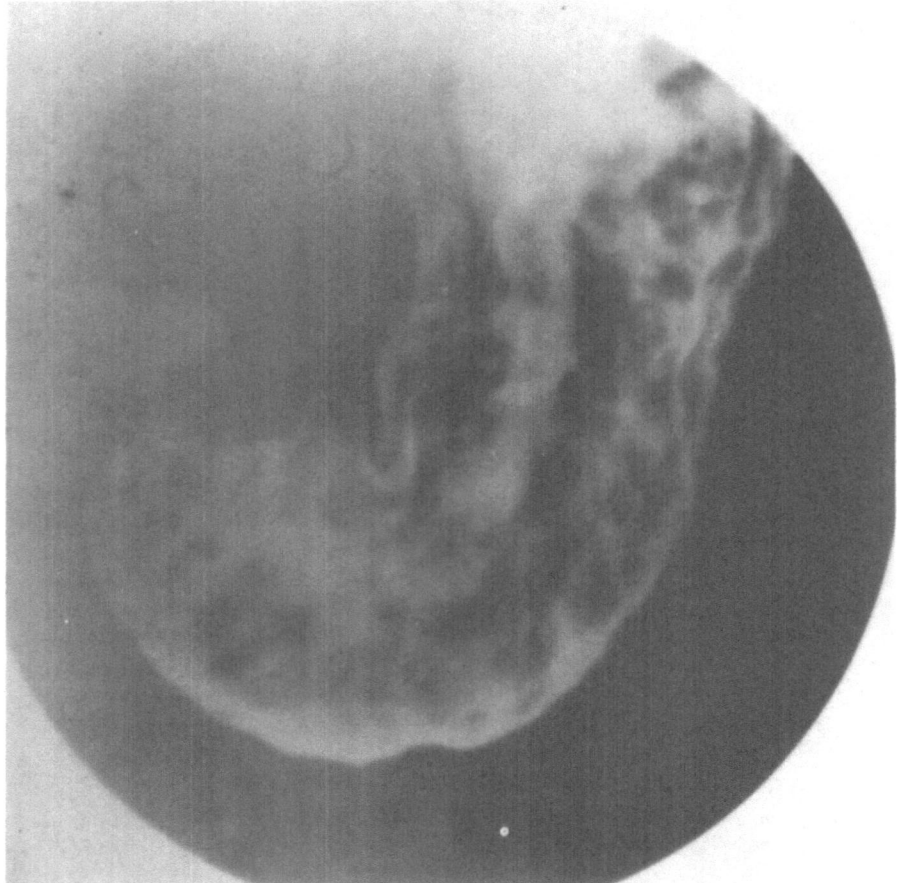

Figure 18-4B Small ulcers are surrounded by edema halo. The ulcers resemble coarse aphthous ulcers of Crohn's disease. Endoscopy confirmed the diagnosis, and the ulcers disappeared on ulcer therapy.

and pouch, or by the antegrade method, allowing the barium to reach the pouch from the proximal small bowel and then introducing air in retrograde fashion for double-contrast study. The retrograde method involves the use of high density barium followed by injection of air through the same tube, thus outlining the mucosa of the pouch, demonstrating an ulcer or fistula, and evaluating the nipple valve with respect to its length, or any degree of deintussusception if difficulty with intubation or incontinence has occurred. The two methods can be combined by aspirating all the ingested barium in the continent ileostomy pouch, and introducing air and high density barium in retrograde fashion.

By choosing the appropriate method, it is possible to investigate fully the ileostomy

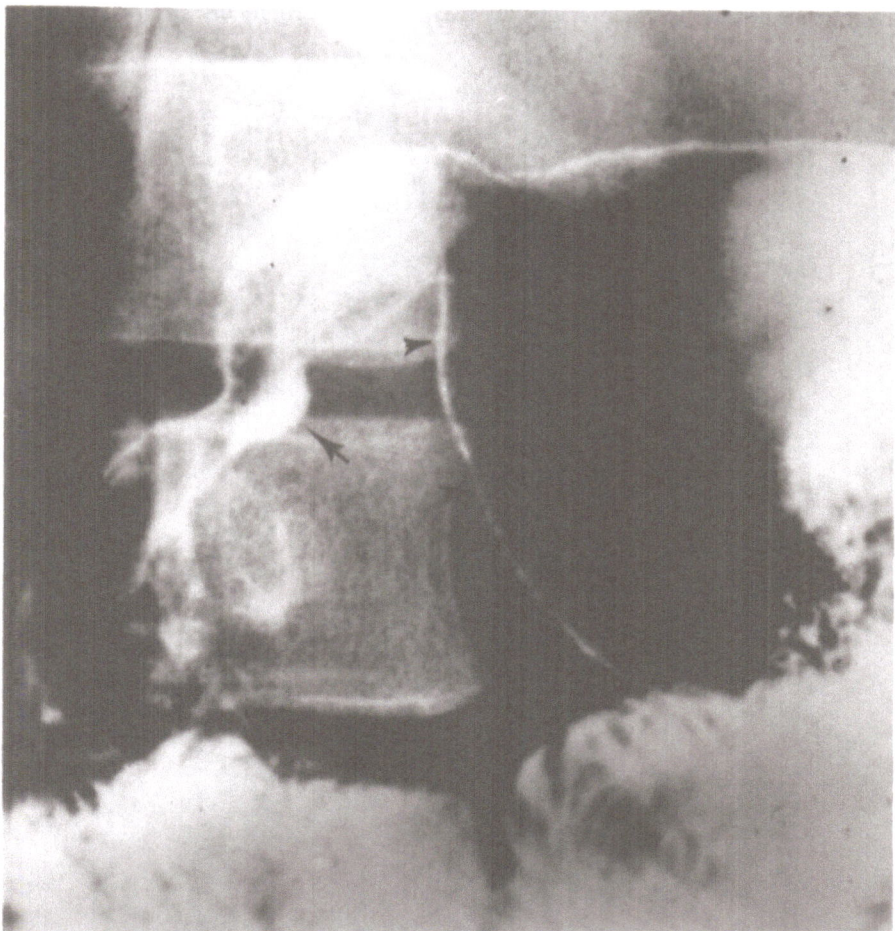

Figure 18-5 Crohn's gastroduodenitis: The antrum of the stomach shows minute ulcerations surrounded by edema halo (aphthous ulcers) along the greater curvature (arrow heads). The pyloric channel is short and patulous with irregular margins due to inflammatory process. The duodenal bulb is shrunken with longitudinal ridging. A smooth, deep ulcer at the apex of the bulb, with tapered narrowing distally and proximally, is rare in Crohn's disease, and could be superimposed peptic ulcer (arrow).

pouch, the nipple valve, and even the efferent loop of the ileostomy, as it traverses the anterior abdominal wall (Figure 18-6).

The newer modalities of investigating IBD in the stomach and duodenum have demonstrated that there is a higher incidence of gastric and duodenal involvement in Crohn's disease, and they have also demonstrated other inflammatory processes in the stomach and duodenum such as erosive gastritis and duodenitis. In the small bowel it has become possible to demonstrate shorter segments of involvement by IBD to demonstrate more clearly sites of chronic obstruction and fistulization and, in some cases, to differentiate inflammatory involvement from neoplasia. Minimal disease in the colon can be more accurately demonstrated by the double-contrast technique. Computerized tomography has been of considerable use in differentiating IBD, especially Crohn's disease or lymphoma.

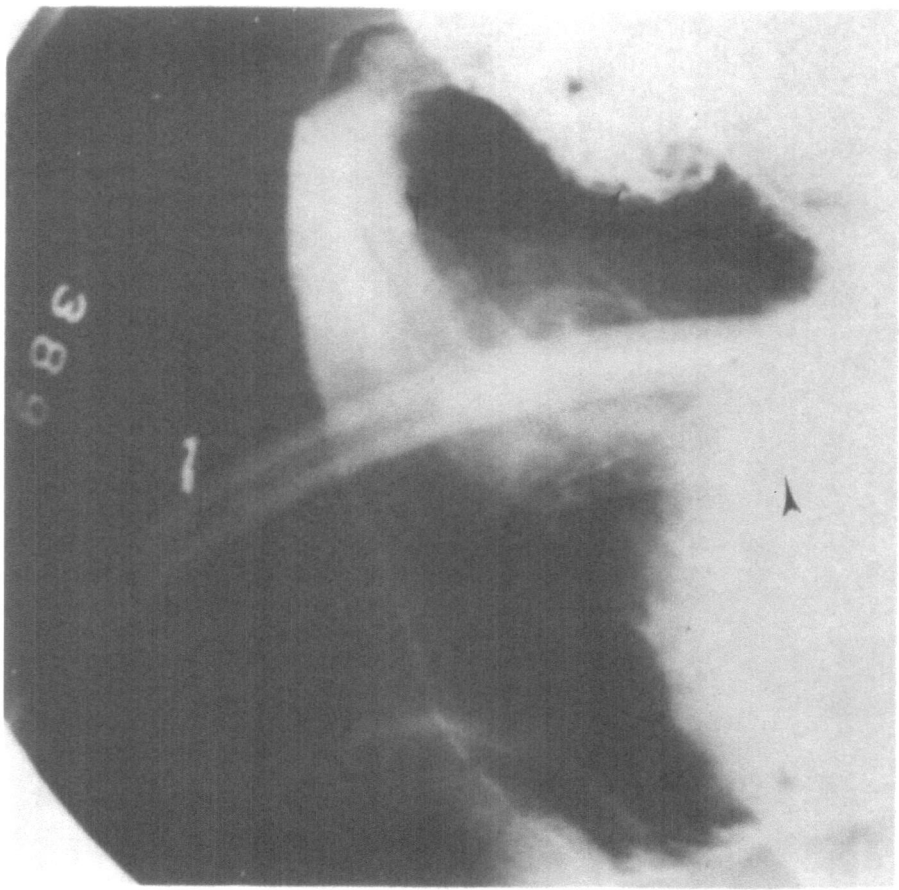

Figure 18-6 Continent ileostomy – double-contrast study: 5 cm-long normal nipple valve is outlined by barium and air in the ileostomy pouch (arrow heads). The drainage tube passes through the nipple valve into the pouch. The lead marker (arrow) is on the skin at the ileostomy stoma. The efferent loop, lying in the anterior abdominal wall, extends from the stoma to the base of the nipple valve.

BIBLIOGRAPHY

Edell SL: Erythema multiforme secondary to intravenous glucagon. *Am J Radiol* 134:385–386, 1980.

Frank PH, Riddell RH, Feczko PJ, et al: Radiological detection of colonic dysplasia (precarcinoma) in chronic ulcerative colitis. *J Gastrointes Radiol* 3:209–219, 1978.

Herlinger H, Laufer I: *Double Contrast Gastrointestinal Radiology.* Philadelphia, WB Saunders Company, 1979, pp 423–494.

Laufer I: *Double Contrast Gastrointestinal Radiology.* Philadelphia, WB Saunders Company, 1979.

Montagne JE, Kressel HY, Moss AA, et al: Radiologic evaluation of continent ileostomy (KOCK). *Radiology* 127:325–329, 1978.

Morson BE, Dawson IMP: *Gastrointestinal Pathology.* London, Blackwell Scientific Publications, 1972, pp 243–298; 448–492.

Sellink JL: *Radiologic Atlas of Common Diseases of the Small Bowel.* Leiden, Stenfert HE, Kroese BV (eds), 1976.

Stephens DH, Mantell BE, Kelly KA: Radiology of the continent ileostomy. *Am J Radiol* 132:717–721, 1979.

19 When in the Course of Crohn's Disease Should X-ray Studies be Performed?

Arthur E. Lindner, MD

One way to consider this matter is to think about managing patients with Crohn's disease from the point of view of the initial diagnostic evaluation, then from the point of view of routine examinations during the course of the patient's illness, and finally the special indications for doing x-ray studies during the course of the patient's illness.

Crohn's disease can involve any part of the gastrointestinal tract and there is no question that x-ray studies are essential in arriving at a diagnosis. The initial studies involve a barium enema, upper gastrointestinal and small bowel examinations. Perhaps the most important point in the initial workup is that positive findings in one area do not exclude disease elsewhere. Thus, an abnormal barium enema showing Crohn's disease does not exclude Crohn's disease involving the duodenum. Another problem in the initial evaluation is the patient who presents with atypical features, one who has few or no gastrointestinal symptoms to lead one to consider Crohn's disease, but who presents with one or more of the extraintestinal manifestations. Patients may present with arthritis or unexplained fever, and children may exhibit only failure to grow. These are patients in whom the gastrointestinal manifestations are lacking. One might not even consider gastrointestinal x-ray studies. Extraintestinal features may dominate the clinical feature but do not change the need for diagnostic x-ray studies.

Usually it is not difficult to make an x-ray diagnosis of Crohn's disease, but at times the findings are equivocal, and sometimes one is not sure whether diagnostic features are present or not. In such cases, repeat studies are necessary at the time of the initial examination.

The final consideration about the initial x-ray studies is the need for distinguishing Crohn's disease from ulcerative colitis. This is important because there is a difference in prognosis and management, and expectations from drug therapy. There is also a difference, especially with respect to carcinoma. The risk of carcinoma in ulcerative colitis may dominate our management of the disease. In Crohn's disease it is a finding of concern, but is not so essential in following patients. The distinction is important if a continent ileostomy is contemplated, since one would not want to perform a continent ileostomy in a patient with Crohn's disease who has a risk of recurrence and loss of additional ileal tissue.

Must everybody have serial examinations during the course of illness that may run 10 years, 20 years, 30 years? There is a difference of opinion about this. It is useful to have x-rays to follow the clinical course of the disease. As far as x-rays are concerned, Crohn's disease tends not to spread linearly within the bowel, but it worsens within the area of involvement. The natural history of the disease includes a tendency toward stenosis. It is helpful in the management of patients to follow that progress and to know at what point in the development of stenosis the patient has reached.

Routine examinations can be of value, but how often? Perhaps every three years would be one way to approach it, not a hard and fast number by any means. Occasionally one can see, instead of the tendency toward stenosis and worsening in the area, the opposite, that is, clinical improvement associated with radiological improvement. This is not a common phenomenon, because usually the x-ray either stays the same or gets worse, but at times, with therapy, the x-ray picture improves. This is an interesting finding to document on films. Postoperatively, routine x-ray examination can be of value. It can determine the length and function of the residual bowel after resection, and can help distinguish postoperative deformities from recurrences. If routine follow-up studies are done, it is apparent that some recurrences that develop after surgery are asymptomatic and will not be detected unless the patient is examined radiologically. It is such asymptomatic recurrences that have demonstrated the high rate of recurrence in Crohn's disease.

During the course of the illness there are special indications for x-ray studies. One of these is the development of intestinal obstruction. X-rays help to determine the site of obstruction, and allow a follow-up of the results of management. In a distended abdomen radiography can differentiate between colonic distention and small bowel obstruction, and assists in determining whether an obstructed bowel is caused by adhesions or inflammatory disease. The development of an abdominal mass is an indication for x-rays to aid in the diagnosis of the nature of the mass. When hydronephrosis is suspected, an intravenous pyelogram is useful, especially in ileocolic lesions and disease of the right side of the abdomen. When fever occurs during the course of Crohn's disease, is it recurrence? Is it increased activity of the disease? What site is involved? X-rays can help. When anemia develops, is it from carcinoma? Is it from recurrent disease? Is it from concurrent disease quite unrelated to Crohn's disease? When hemorrhage occurs, and massive bleeding can occur in Crohn's disease, is the bleeding from the disease? If so, where? Or is it from some other disease, such as a peptic ulcer? When a patient has lost weight and the weight loss cannot be explained during the course of the illness, has an internal fistula developed? Finally, when a patient had disease at a stoma, what is the explanation? Is it recurrent disease? Is it ileostomy dysfunction? X-ray can be of help in making such distinctions. The indications for radiography in Crohn's disease are summarized in Table 19-1.

Table 19-1
When in the Course of Crohn's Disease Should X-rays be Performed?

A. Initial diagnostic evaluation

1. Any area of bowel may be involved. Initial studies include barium enema, upper gastrointestinal series, small bowel examination. Positive findings in one area do not exclude disease elsewhere.
2. High index of suspicion required in patients with unusual presentations—eg, arthritis, unexplained fever, failure of growth in children—in absence of gastrointestinal symptoms. Extraintestinal features may dominate clinical picture.
3. Repeat studies may be required if initial examination is equivocal, either for presence of disease or for differential diagnosis. Usually, x-ray findings in Crohn's disease are not subtle or difficult.
4. Importance of distinguishing Crohn's colitis from ulcerative colitis: difference in prognosis and management, especially with respect to risk of carcinoma; essential distinction if continent ileostomy is contemplated.

B. Routine examinations during course of illness

1. Follow progress of disease: it tends not to spread but to worsen and progress toward stenosis. Recommended routine frequency of examination varies—perhaps every three years.
2. Occasional dramatic improvement on therapy.
3. Postoperative assessment of length and function of residual bowel; postoperative deformities vs recurrence. Asymptomatic recurrence.

C. Special indications for radiography during course of illness

1. Intestinal obstruction: a) site of obstruction and follow-up for management; b) colonic dilatation vs small bowel obstruction; c) adhesions vs inflammatory disease.
2. Development of an abdominal mass
   Nature of the mass
   Intravenous pyelogram—hydronephrosis?
3. Development of fever. Recurrence? Activity of disease? What site?
4. Development of anemia. Carcinoma? Concurrent disease?
5. Development of hemorrhage from Crohn's or concurrent disease, eg, peptic ulcer.
6. Development of unexplained weight loss. Internal fistula?
7. Evaluation of stomal disease: ileostomy dysfunction vs Crohn's disease.

BIBLIOGRAPHY

Davidson M: Medical treatment and prognosis of ulcerative colitis and Crohn's disease in children. In *Inflammatory Bowel Disease,* Kirsner JB, Shorter RG (eds).

Philadelphia, Lea & Febiger, 1975, pp 310–312.

Marshak RH: Granulomatous disease of the intestinal tract. *Radiology* 114:3–22, 1975.

Marshak RH, Lindner AE: *Radiology of the Small Intestine.* 2nd Ed. Philadelphia, Saunders, 1976, pp 179–300.

Marshak RH, Lindner AE, Maklansky D: *Radiology of the Colon.* Philadelphia, Saunders, 1980, pp 120–188.

PANEL DISCUSSION

Moderator: Burton I. Korelitz, MD

Queston: How often are granulomas found in skip lesions? Are skip lesions found in all cases?

Dr Rotterdam: We know that some cases of Crohn's disease never develop granulomas and we do not know why that is so. I think there are many open questions and I do not really have an answer.

Dr Korelitz: In addition to skip areas grossly and macroscopically, Dr Sommers has reported skip lesions histologically. That occurred in a recent case.

Dr Rickert: We found microgranulomas and fully developed ones at the base of the ulcers adjacent to them. I think they are probably the ulcerative lesion, although that is hard to confirm. It may be that the ulcers can occur in tissue other than a granuloma.

Question: Does the finding of an aphthoid lesion in normal mucosa after surgical resection signify recurrence or earlier involvement?

Dr Korelitz: It is a very practical clinical question but has there been a clinical application of that, Dr Rickert?

Dr Rickert: Not to my knowledge. When we are considering these earlier ulcerative lesions, one must keep in mind that these are being seen in the same surgical specimens which harbor what we would consider advanced disease. During the second 30 some cases that we have looked at, some of our initial cases have had an opportunity to recur. Although our numbers have not yet been tabulated with a second study, I have the feeling that those cases initially seen with the largest number of aphthoid lesions are the ones that are recurring. At least, all of those patients who are now contributing the second and third specimens to our study had aphthoid lesions rather easily seen initially.

Dr Korelitz: Of course, the practical implication of your question is in the hands of the surgeon, in a sense, who for years has meticulously examined both ends of the surgical specimen to decide whether he has taken enough tissue without ever having known whether it made any difference or not. So, even if we found those aphthoid lesions proximal to the line of resection, it is questionable whether it should lead to a more extensive resection.

Question: Do you have any experience with cases in which the only means of diagnosis of Crohn's disease was an abnormal rectal biopsy with everything else normal?

Dr Korelitz: We had such a case recently in a woman who was being studied for diarrhea of undetermined origin. Her x-rays were absolutely normal and the rectal biopsy showed Crohn's disease.

Question: With normal mucosa at sigmoidoscopy, how often is a biopsy diagnosis of Crohn's disease possible?

Dr Sommers: In sigmoidoscopically normal mucosa, McGovern in Australia, and also our series, were 30% diagnostic for Crohn's disease.

Question Dr Korelitz, what kind of biopsy forceps do you use and from where do you take the biopsy? Is there any significant difference between specimens obtained in colonoscopic and sigmoidoscopic biopsies?

Dr Korelitz: I will answer only the first part of the question. I use a punch biopsy forceps, not the suction type, and if the tissue is normal or representative throughout the whole distance of the sigmoidoscopy, I then take the biopsy from as far distally as possible, mostly to reduce the risk of bleeding that cannot be controlled. If the mucosa appears normal, I sometimes take the biopsy at a valve because that is through-and-through, mucosa-to-mucosa. Often, if the mucosa is loose enough, I might take it from an area even more distal than that. If there is a representative lesion, that is different.

Question: Are any special methods used for preparing microscopic slides of rectal or endoscopic biopsies?

Dr Sommers: We do not impose any restrictions or special requirements on the clinicians. There are so many different methods. Technicians seem to be able to orient the specimens so that the sections are perpendicular to the surface. We do use Bouin's fixative. We think it gives a little better cell detail than formalin and a little brighter staining. We use a trichrome stain for all surgical specimens, not just for rectal biopsies.

Dr Korelitz: The rest of the question concerns the difference between the rectal biopsy and the colonoscopic biopsy.

Dr Sommers: We do not have any restrictions on colonoscopic biopsies. They arrive as the person wants to send them in. Some places use Gelfoam with the raw surface attached to the Gelfoam. The endoscopist or colonoscopist is allowed to put them on filter paper or leave them floating in the fixative. That is all right. They are labeled A through Z and processed that way.

Dr Korelitz: In general, do they prove to be as valuable as rectal biopsies?

Dr Sommers: Dr Waye obtains a "bigger bite" and more representative biopsy than the inexperienced colonoscopist. In general, they are as difficult to learn to interpret as fiberoptic bronchoscopic biopsies have been in the last few years. The volume of the sample and the possible sampling area are potentially of greater value in rectal biopsies than small bronchoscopic or colonoscopic biopsies.

Dr Korelitz: My own bias in answer to the question, influenced by the reports from Dr Sommers and Dr Rotterdam, is that more information can be obtained from the rectal biopsies, which are bigger and deeper in general than the colonoscopic biopsies. Of course, the latter cover a far greater extent of the disease.

Question: Were any immunologic studies done on the Crohn's disease biopsies?

Dr Rotterdam: The only immunologic studies we have done are on the plasma cell population around granulomas. Other investigators have done the same thing. This is a polymorphous infiltrate of IGG-, IGM-, and IGA-producing plasma cells, but in very distinct proportions. We have not studied granulomas themselves, and I do not know of anybody else who has studied them by immunofluorescence.

Dr Rickert: We have done a few of the aphthoid lesions. It is a real exercise, technically, to try to dissect out a lesion that is a millimeter or two in diameter at the most — generally much smaller. We tried a variety of techniques to do direct immuno-fluorescent staining, mainly to try to get some display of the T and B cell populations at the base of the ulcers. So far, in the few specimens we have done, we have not noted any significant difference in the lymphoid tissue away from those ulcers, but this is a very preliminary finding. Direct immunofluorescent staining is undergoing many changes. We are now able to use some techniques with fixed tissue and obtain a more easily oriented specimen, so that one is quite confident that one is looking at immunofluo-rescence, which can be superimposed on light microscopy. So far there has been no meaningful information. We have looked at them, and they are pretty, but we do not know what they mean.

Question: I would like to ask Dr Rickert: Is the intestinal inflammatory reaction to *Yersinia* at all similar to inflammatory bowel disease in the aphthoid lesions that you have observed?

Dr Rickert: In the one case where we were able to discover what we thought were very early *Yersinia* lesions, the very early reaction was a necrotizing pustular reaction rather than the kind seen in Crohn's disease. It was intriguing that the early lesions had the same orientation in terms of their relationship to lymphoid tissue as the typical lesions in Crohn's disease. If the etiologic agent in *Yersinia* can attack a single lymphoid follicle and the organisms can divide there and be recognized both by conventional histologic staining for bacteria and by electronmicroscopy, that might be a good place to look. The tissue reaction is not the same. It is just the localization in the relationship of the early lesion to lymphoid tissue which is quite similar.

Dr Korelitz: Does anybody disagree with Dr Lindner on the frequency of x-ray procedures in Crohn's disease? Should we always wait for symptoms or should the x-rays be done routinely and more frequently?

Question: Are you concerned about the amount of radiation to which the patient is exposed when x-rays are done routinely?

Dr Lindner: Of course, this is of concern, and one must restrict the amount of radiation. Some small bowel series, for example, can continue with multiple spot views and an enormous amount of radiation, so that radiation must be minimized. In a patient who has a chronic illness like Crohn's disease, three years is not an inordinate risk to the patient. Most of the time, x-rays will be done for specific indications during that period of time.

Dr Korelitz: I am a little more aggressive than that. I feel that there is some risk every three years and a greater risk every year, but I would still aim toward a little bit earlier than three years. I have seen many cases where the changes have been insidious and not accompanied by symptoms, and if I had seen the progressive development of a stricture earlier, I might have treated the patient more aggressively. I, too, respect the matter of radiation and cancer but this is a terrible disease and one risk must be weighed against the other.

Question: Are lymphoid follicles limited to Crohn's disease?

Dr Sohn: This question sounds very familiar. We see it in Crohn's disease, in nonspecific proctitis, in the classical ulcerative proctitis and we also see it in proctitis of other etiologies, particularly nonspecific proctitis in male homosexuals, which resolves with no specific therapy. We have biopsied these cases and received reports of lymphoid follicles. I tend to think that this is a resolving phase of proctitis.

Dr Korelitz: Could you add anything to that, Dr Rotterdam?

Dr Rotterdam: Lymphoid follicles are, of course, one of the histologic features seen in the mucosa, submucosa, and serosa, but if you have a mucosal biopsy and the only abnormality is an increase in lymphoid tissue, I do not think that is diagnostic of anything. Many of our cases showed lymphoid follicles besides granulomas and other changes, but by themselves these do not help to make a specific diagnosis.

PART IV

Moderator: Felicien M. Steichen, MD

20 Recurrence Rates After Surgery for Crohn's Disease and Their Implications Regarding Indications for Surgery (As Seen by the Gastroenterologist)

Burton I. Korelitz, MD

The history of surgery is very important in order to understand the best total management of the disease. This chapter is limited to Crohn's disease and does not include ulcerative colitis.

Table 20-1 shows some statistics on surgery and mortality in Crohn's disease. The incidence of surgical intervention in ileitis has changed very little, being approximately 60%. In other words, given enough time, about 60% of patients with ileitis are going to come to surgery. The mortality has decreased significantly in the past few decades, but the surgical incidence has remained about the same. In two large studies of Crohn's colitis, done at two different periods of time, the surgical incidence has remained about 40%, but the mortality has been much less than with ileitis. This too appears to have decreased since the early years.

With colitis in the elderly, the surgical incidence has been much higher and the mortality has been reduced considerably in recent years since this entity has been recognized. However, we still know very little about inflammatory bowel disease (IBD) in the elderly.

Table 20-2 shows recurrence rates after surgery for Crohn's disease, based on studies

125

Table 20-1
Surgery and Mortality in Crohn's Disease

Extent of Disease	Years Concerned	Total No. of Patients*	Years Followed†	Major Surgery		Mortality*		Comments
				No.	%	No.	%	
All	1931–1968	295	14	199	57	33	11	Cumulative
	1939–1968	332	30	81	88	11	3	
	1960–1968	92	17	25	29	0	9	
	1966–1976	86	6				0	Children
Ileitis	1929–1960	168	1–34	147	87	16	10	Mostly aged
	1939–1968	136	30	283	58		2	
	1961–1970		1–26				10	Surgical cases only
Ileocolitis	1928–1947	75	1–19	55	73		16	
	1934–1962		1–10	172	most	20	12	
	1939–1968	115	30		64		4	Mostly aged
	1952–1961	94	14	68	72		12	Worse with involvement of terminal ileum
Ileocolitis and colitis	1936–1964	25	17	17	68	17	16	Children
	1938–1970	221	9		74		8	
Colitis	1939–1968	70	30		47		4	
	1952–1971		8	64		8	12	Surgical cases only
Left-sided colitis	1952–1972	80	34	33	41		3	Mostly aged
	1952–1972	26	7	26			0	Surgical cases only

*Figures modified from original for adequate follow-up and death actually due to Crohn's disease when necessary information available.
†Mean, average, or range.

Table 20-2
Recurrence Rates After Surgery for Crohn's Disease

Extent of Disease	Operative Procedure	Recurrence Rate (%)	Time Postoperative Mean or Range (yrs)
Ileitis	Bypass and continuity	87	
		92	
		89	5
		90	11
		61	5
	Resection and internal anastomosis	50	
		18	5
		43	5
		51	10
		40	
		50	10
		37	5
		80	1–26
		69	3.3
Ileitis or ileocolitis	Bypass and continuity	100	
		82	
	Resection and internal anastomosis	100	17 (children)
		74	
		50	
		71	
		60	
		40	
		34	5
		77	1–26 (children)
Ileocolitis or colitis	Resection and internal anastomosis	47	
		84	
		75	
		50	
		45	
		12	
		50	
		18	1
		64	
	Ileostomy and resection	20	
		52	
		11	1–10
		15	5–19 (based on resected specimens)
		46	7
		0	5.5
		17	10–17
		10–12	12.8
		33	8.7
		31	8.6
		28	13.1 (based on resected specimens)
		60	6 (children)
		7.4	
		8	10–17
		28	9 (young patients)
		5.7	

Table 20-2
Recurrence Rates After Surgery for Crohn's Disease *(continued)*

Extent of Disease	Operative Procedure	Recurrence Rate (%)	Time Postoperative Mean or Range (yrs)
Colitis	Ileostomy or colostomy alone	3/4	1
		17/19	1
		0	16 mos
		15/29	1
Left-sided colitis	Colostomy and resection	4/45	1
		1/12	
		1/24	7.3
		4/7	9 mos

performed over a period of many years. When bypass and continuity has been done for ileitis, recurrence rates have varied from 61% to 92%. The results have been somewhat better with resection and anastomosis. In studies which included a combination of ileitis and ileocolitis, there was up to 100% recurrence with bypass and continuity, and from 34% to 100% recurrence in patients with resection and anastomosis if they were followed long enough. In ileitis or colitis after resection and anastomosis, the recurrence rate has been considerably less in some series, ranging from 12% to 84%. When ileostomy has been performed for Crohn's colitis or ileocolitis, the recurrence rate after ileostomy has been reported as ranging from 0% to 66%. With colitis alone, the recurrence rate after ileostomy or colostomy ranges from 0% to 90%. Left-sided colitis treated by colostomy and resection has been reported as low as 4% and as high as 57%.

One thing learned from cumulative studies of recurrence rates following surgery for Crohn's disease is that the disease at onset under age 25 is more virulent. Following resection, the recurrence occurs earlier than in the older age groups. Contrary to what was once thought to be the case, following one resection for Crohn's disease, the likelihood of a recurrence keeps increasing with each subsequent resection rather than decreasing.

Formerly, the most common operation performed was a side-to-side ileotransverse colostomy, and the recurrence occurred in the afferent loop. When an end-to-end anastomosis became the most popular procedure, again the recurrence was in the ileum, just proximal to the anastomosis. An ileostomy performed for diffuse Crohn's disease of the colon provides no protection against proximal spread of the disease.

In our study at Mount Sinai Hospital, we followed 31 cases of recurrent ileitis in the ileostomy following colectomy for Crohn's colitis or ileocolitis. In 14 cases, a single ileal resection was later required. Six cases required multiple ileal resections. Eight patients had such extensive recurrence that resection was no longer possible. They were crippled by the disease and three patients died of recurrent ileitis. Therefore, recurrent ileitis with ileostomy is a potentially incapacititating disease.

With regard to the mortality and morbidity in the 31 cases of recurrent ileitis, two died from fulminating disease, eight were treated medically with steroids for extended periods, six were crippled by multiple resections and complications including short bowel syndromes, recurrent obstructions, intermittent bleeding, abscesses, uric acid uropathy, and postnecrotic cirrhosis.

In Goligher's most recent study of ileostomy and total colectomy for Crohn's disease, his figures approach ours. After 15 to 18 years of follow-up, the recurrence rate was 43%.

Given enough time, the recurrence following surgery for Crohn's disease approaches 100%, occurring earliest after bypass operations, then after resections with anastomosis, and least after ileostomy or colostomy. "The least" means that recurrence occurs later in time, but it still occurs. It is seen earlier in proportion to the extent of the disease. This means that if the ileitis is extensive initially, requiring surgery, recurrence is likely to occur earlier, less likely after a more localized ileitis or ileocolitis, still less after a limited colitis, and the very least after a left-sided colitis or disease limited to the anorectal area.

Recurrence is more common in young people than in older people because the former have a more virulent form of disease. Recurrences occur later in old people. The indication for the original operation does not appear to play any role in the recurrence rate, but the nature of the recurrence usually is similar to the nature of the original disease process prior to resection. The duration of the disease before the surgery does not appear to be a factor. The fact that the margins are free of disease in the resected specimen has not really proven over a long period of time to be an advantage in monitoring or preventing the recurrence. Finally, the risk increases with successive operations.

A long time ago, a list of indications for surgical intervention was headed by perirectal suppuration. In an earlier study there were 11 cases of perirectal suppuration and 9 cases of abdominal mass and fistulae; these accounted for more than 50% of the indications. Today the indications for surgery are vastly modified.

In considering the indications for surgery, one must think in terms of how severe the disease is in the first place, what complications are present, what was the original extent of involvement, the anticipated extension in both directions, and how much time it might take until that extension takes place. The quality of life between surgical resections must also be considered, provided resection was initially considered.

In our recent studies with mercaptopurine, we have been able to close perirectal fistulae in 50% and abdominal wall fistulae in 83% of cases. My own current attitude about indications for surgery are divided into three groups. Absolute indications include free perforation, massive hemorrhage, possible appendicitis, and carcinoma of the ileum or colon.

Relative indications include: 1) small bowel obstruction, which can be relieved completely followed by long-term medical therapy; 2) intraabdominal abscesses, using combination therapy including antibiotics, with subsequent long-term medical therapy; 3) perirectal fistulae and abscesses; 4) toxic megacolon, which is reversible in the majority of cases; 5) blind loop syndrome, which can be treated medically; 6) retarded growth and development, for which total parenteral nutrition and enforced elemental nutrition have been shown to reverse the trend and even lead to growth acceleration; 7) rectal incontinence; 8) chronic obstruction and malabsorption, which may at times be reversed with intensive, sustained medical therapy; and 9) hydroureter and hydronephrosis, which often require surgery.

Infrequent indications for surgery include: 1) intraabdominal fistulae, provided they do not cause symptoms and which can be treated medically; 2) multiple perineal fistulae, which often heal with immunosuppressive therapy or metronidazole; 3) abdominal wall fistulae, which respond to mercaptopurine in about 80% of cases; 4) colonic strictures, which should be left alone if there is no fear of carcinoma; and 5) a nontender abdominal mass, which usually disappears with concentrated effort.

Rectovaginal fistulae should never be treated surgically. Recurrent ileitis and extraintestinal manifestations can be treated medically, the latter with steroids.

BIBLIOGRAPHY

Alexander-Williams J, Fielding J, Cooke WT: A comparison of results of excision and bypass for ileal Crohn's disease. *Gut* 13:973–975, 1972.

Atwell JD, Duthie HL, Goligher JC: The outcome of Crohn's disease. *Br J Surg* 52:966–972, 1965.

Baker WNW: Ileo-rectal anastomosis for Crohn's disease of the colon. *Gut* 12:427–431, 1971.

Banks BM, Zetzel L, Richter HS: Morbidity and mortality in regional enteritis. *Am J Dig Dis* 14:369–379, 1969.

Brill CB, Klein SF, Kark AE: Regional enteritis and entero-colitis. *Ann Surg* 170:166–174, 1969.

Burman JH, Cooke WT, Alexander-Williams J: The fate of ileorectal anastomosis in Crohn's disease. *Gut* 12:432–436, 1971.

Colcock BP, Vansant JH: Surgical treatment of regional enteritis. *N Engl J Med* 262:435–439, 1960.

Cornes JS, Stecker M: Primary Crohn's disease of the colon and rectum. *Gut* 2:189–201, 1961.

Crohn BB, Garlock JH, Yarni SH: Right sided (regional) colitis. *JAMA* 135:334–338, 1954.

deDombal FT, Burton IL, Goligher JC: Recurrence of Crohn's disease after primary excisional surgery. *Gut* 12:519–527, 1971.

deDombal FT, Burton IL, Clamp SE, et al: Short term course and prognosis of Crohn's disease. *Gut* 15:435–443, 1974.

Fawaz KA, Glotzer DJ, Goldman H, et al: Ulcerative colitis and Crohn's disease of the colon – a comparison of the long term postoperative courses. *Gastroenterology* 71:372–378, 1976.

Fromm H, Wilson FA, Rodgers JB Jr, et al: Granulomatous bowel (Crohn's) disease. *Arch Intern Med* 128:739–745, 1971.

Glotzer DJ, Gardner RC, Goldman H, et al: Comparative features and course of ulcerative and granulomatous colitis. *N Engl J Med* 282:582–587, 1970.

Gryboski JD, Spiro HM: Prognosis in children with Crohn's disease. *Gastroenterology* 74:807–817, 1978.

Hawk WA, Turnbull RB Jr: Primary ulcerative disease of the colon. *Gastroenterology* 51:802–805, 1966.

Jones JH, Lennard-Jones JE, Lockhart-Mummery HH: Experience in the treatment of Crohn's disease of the large intestine. *Gut* 7:448–452, 1966.

Korelitz BI: Clinical course, late results and pathological nature of inflammatory disease of the colon initially sparing the rectum. *Gut* 8:281–290, 1967.

Korelitz BI, Gribetz D, Kopel FB: Granulomatous colitis in children: a study of 25 cases and comparisons with ulcerative colitis. *Pediatrics* 42:446–457, 1968.

Korelitz BI, Present DH, Alpert LI, et al: Recurrent regional ileitis after ileostomy and colectomy for granulomatous colitis. *N Engl J Med* 287:110–115, 1972.

Lennard-Jones JE, Stalder GA: Prognosis after resection of chronic regional ileitis. *Gut* 8:332–336, 1967.

Lockhart-Mummery HH: Crohn's disease of the large bowel. *Br J Surg* 59:823–826, 1972.

Nugent FW, Veidenheimer MC, Meissner WA, et al: Prognosis after colonic resection for Crohn's disease of the colon. *Gastroenterology* 65:398–401, 1973.

Prior P, Fielding JF, Waterhouse JA, et al: Mortality in Crohn's disease. *Lancet* 1:1135–1137, 1970.

Ritchie JK, Lockhart-Mummery HH: Non-restorative surgery in the treatment of Crohn's disease of the large bowel. *Gut* 14:263–269, 1973.

Ritchie JK, Lennard-Jones JE: Crohn's disease of the distal large bowel. *Scand J Gastroenterol* 11:433–436, 1976.

Schofield PF: The natural history and treatment of Crohn's disease. *Ann R Coll Surg Engl* 36:258–279, 1965.

Steinberg DM, Allan RH, Thompson H, et al: Excisional surgery with ileostomy for Crohn's disease with particular reference to factors affecting recurrence. *Gut* 15:845–851, 1974.

Stone W, Veidenheimer MC, Gorman ML, et al: The dilemma of Crohn's disease: long-term follow-up of Crohn's disease of the small intestine. *Dis Colon Rectum* 26:372–376, 1977.

Truelove SC, Pena AS: Course and prognosis of Crohn's disease. *Gut* 17:192–201, 1976.

Veidenheimer MC, Nugent FW, Haggitt RC: Differentiation between chronic ulcerative colitis and Crohn's colitis. *Surg Clin North Am* 56:722–726, 1976.

Weterman IT, Pena AS: The long-term prognosis of ileorectal anastomosis and proctocolectomy in Crohn's disease. *Scand J Gastroenterol* 11:185–191, 1976.

Young S, Smith IS, O'Connor J, et al: Results of surgery for Crohn's disease in the Glasgow region. *Br J Surg* 62:528–534, 1975.

21 Indications for Surgery in Crohn's Disease (As Seen by the Colon and Rectal Surgeon)

Norman Sohn, MD

The decision to offer an operation to a patient with Crohn's disease is tempered by the inordinately high recurrence rate. Indeed, there are those who believe that any bowel operation in Crohn's disease will increase the possibility of a recurrence. The indications for emergency surgery are often catastrophic and clear-cut. The indication for elective surgery may be more subtle and subjective. Crohn's disease is a disease of unknown etiology and is incurable by treatment available today. The surgeon, particularly, should not expect to cure the disease. Surgery should rather be directed toward palliating symptoms and improving the patient's lifestyle. Surgery should not be viewed as an isolated event in the management of the patient with Crohn's disease, but should be integrated as part of a comprehensive program including medical therapy and nutritional support.

The indications for emergency surgery are hemorrhage, a severe acute attack, toxic megacolon, or perforation. These may represent a common condition of varying severity.

The close interplay of medical and surgical therapy is particularly reflected in the management of these conditions. Obviously, perforation is an indication for immediate surgery. With hemorrhage, a severe acute attack, or toxic megacolon, the patient should be offered a trial of intensive medical therapy, including the use of corticosteroids or

ACTH, total parenteral nutrition (TPN), and possibly the use of albumin, antibiotics or a long intestinal tube, along with close monitoring of the patient, frequent examination, and x-rays at least daily. Hemorrhage does not usually occur so rapidly that the patient cannot be readily resuscitated with adequate blood transfusions. This is unlike upper gastrointestinal bleeding such as occurs from a duodenal ulcer, in which a major vessel may be the source of bleeding, and in which surgical control of the bleeding site is an essential part of resuscitation. The bleeding rate in Crohn's disease is usually such that adequate blood replacement can easily be accomplished and give the surgeon adequate time to improve the patient's preoperative condition while offering a trial of medical therapy. Of course, a rapidly exsanguinating type of hemorrhage, for which blood replacement cannot be maintained adequately, would be an indication for urgent surgery. The severe attack and toxic megacolon with no perforation should be managed medically for at least 48 hours. During that time, continuous reevaluation and reassessment can be made. If the condition appears to be exacerbating, surgery is indicated. If the patient is stable or improving, surgery may be safely deferred. Perforation, of course, is an indication for immediate operation.

The basic criterion for elective surgery is improvement in the patient's overall physiologic status. The common indication, which is given as failure of medical therapy, is a very subjective criterion. Failure of medical therapy should be defined as persistence of serious symptoms despite intensive medical therapy, usually, at least in part, on an in-hospital basis, with all reasonable modalities of medical therapy including corticosteroids, ACTH, sulfasalazine, immunosuppressive agents, and TPN. Medical therapy in some patients may be limited due to intolerance to some of these modalities. These patients may be considered for earlier operation. Persistent diarrhea, anemia, hypoproteinemia, or malnutrition, despite intensive medical therapy, suggest the need for operation. Chronic systemic manifestations, such as erythema nodosum, pyoderma gangrenosum, uveitis, or iritis, which fail to respond to medical therapy, are indications for surgery. Most of these can be effectively managed medically. Hepatic problems, including sclerosing cholangitis and biliary cirrhosis, or ankylosing spondylitis, are often not affected by bowel resection.

Growth retardation is often an indication for surgery in a youngster. In this situation, a trial of medical therapy should be offered, but it must be tempered by the knowledge that time may be lost if the surgery is delayed. When appropriate surgical therapy is performed, one may expect an appreciable weight gain, a spurt in growth, and the appearance of normal sexual development in those patients who have reached the age of puberty without normal sexual development. The operation should not be delayed beyond the age of epiphyseal closure.

Intestinal obstruction due to Crohn's disease is an indication for medical therapy along with the use of a long intestinal tube. Prognostically, the development of intestinal obstruction usually indicates that surgery is likely to be necessary in the near future. This is not inevitable, however. The indications for treating intestinal fistulae are dependent on the site of the fistula, the structure with which it communicates, and its physiologic effects. Many will respond to the use of immunosuppressive agents, and some to TPN. The basic criterion of improvement of the patient's physiologic status is particularly relevant here. Enterocutaneous fistulae draining small quantities may be easily managed medically. Higher-volume fistulae which do not cause fluid or electrolyte disorders and in which the fistula's drainage can be collected with no skin irritation, may not represent any physiologic threat to the patient. These fistulae usually occur in patients who have had previous surgery, and reoperation may be difficult and hazardous. It may be advantageous not to operate on the fistula, teach the patient to care for it, and continue medical therapy. The mere presence of a fistula is not an indication for surgery. A high-volume fistula, or one which is particularly proximal in the gastrointestinal tract, or which may interfere with the patient's nutrition, or which may be responsible for unmanageable skin irritation, would be an indication for operative intervention.

Enterovesical fistulae which cause urinary tract infection or renal impairment should be treated surgically. The patient who is tolerating this type of fistula satisfactorily without infection or renal impairment may be offered a trial of medical therapy. Ileosigmoid or ileorectal fistulae occur quite commonly, and these fistulae alone should not be an indication for operation. When surgery is performed on a patient with such a fistula, the diseased segment usually is primary in the ileum, and the ileum often can be dissected off the sigmoid without resecting the latter. There are cases, however, in which this cannot be safely accomplished, and an ileocolic resection as well as a sigmoid resection must be performed. Enterovaginal fistulae usually are quite symptomatic and often require surgery.

An abdominal mass in a patient with Crohn's disease is an indication for medical therapy, not surgery. Resolution of the mass with appropriate medical therapy is hoped for. The presence of an abscess would be suspect in the patient with a mass, particularly if it is associated with fever and abdominal pain. These patients should be treated medically as resolution can occur. The abscess may resolve on medical therapy or may spontaneously drain into the bowel. Failure of resolution of a suspected abscess would lead to an operation. Segmental colon resection should be performed when appropriate. This consists of an ileal or ileocolic resection for disease confined to the ileum or right colon. This can be performed with an anastomosis between the ileum and the ascending or transverse colon. Segmental left colon resections for disease of the sigmoid or descending colon or splenic flexure can be performed. It should be ascertained that there is no residual disease or minimal disease in the segments to be anastomosed. An ileorectal anastomosis can be performed when there is colonic disease with sparing of the rectum. This operation appears to have been more popular a few years ago. The very high recurrence rate with this operation has caused it to lose popularity in many centers. The patient should be prepared to accept the possibility of a subsequent reoperation and subsequent ileostomy. An ileorectal anastomosis is particularly attractive for a young patient in whom it is hoped to postpone an ileostomy for a period of time. In acute ileitis, the surgery is usually being performed on a mistaken diagnosis that the patient has an acute appendicitis. The surgeon is confronted with an acutely inflamed ileum. At this time the appendix should be removed if the cecum appears to be normal. The ileum should not be resected and the patient should be treated medically. While the literature shows that a high percentage of these cases of acute ileitis are unrelated to Crohn's disease, many of these patients go on to develop typical Crohn's ileitis.

Other local rectal operations can be performed in an effort to obviate the need for resection and stoma. Incontinence in Crohn's disease is due either to poorly performed surgery or to progressive rectal suppuration. Fecal incontinence in Crohn's disease can be treated by insertion of a Thiersch wire. In this operation, a stainless steel wire is placed in the perianal tissues to encircle the rectum. This involves minimal dissection and is thus not associated with large perianal wounds which are prone to poor healing. Other operations for incontinence, including sphincterplasties, are contraindicated on this basis. The Thiersch procedure has resulted in improved continuence in this setting.

In general, we discourage the excision of external hemorrhoids. We have successfully ligated internal hemorrhoids which have caused symptoms or protrusion with rubber bands. In general, we prefer not to treat hemorrhoids in patients with Crohn's disease. Most anal fissures in Crohn's disease are painless. The presence of pain should make one suspicious of an underlying abscess. However, fissures can be very painful themselves. Those which fail to respond to medical therapy can be treated by means of a lateral, subcutaneous internal anal sphincterotomy performed through an incision approximately one-quarter inch long. An unhealed one-quarter inch wound is a reasonable price to pay for relief of pain, and healing of these wounds has not been a problem. Occasionally, one sees an unhealed perineal wound in a patient who has had a previous abdominal perineal resection and a proctocolectomy. This can be a very frustrating and difficult problem. These have been treated initially by irrigation with a Water Pik modified for use on the perineum. Those which fail to respond are treated by excision of the wound and its surrounding dense fibrotic tissue. This is sufficient to facilitate healing in some patients. Those that persist despite these maneuvers are treated by excision of the perineal wound and insertion of a gracilis muscle flap. Unhealed perineal wounds which have been present for over ten years have fully resolved by means of this operation.

In summary, the indications for surgery as seen by a colorectal surgeon should be very similar to those seen by the gastroenterologist. There is no operation which can cure Crohn's disease. The spectre of a recurrence looms over the physician contemplating an operation for the Crohn's disease sufferer. The goal of the surgeon is to improve the patient's physiologic status. The surgery must be part of a comprehensive plan which integrates medical therapy and nutritional support.

22 What is the Best Management of Perirectal Abscess and Fistula in Crohn's Disease?

Michael A. Weinstein, MD

The patient suffering from the ravages of anorectal Crohn's disease often has pain, discharge, loss of muscle substance secondary to recurrent abscess, and eventually incontinence. When these patients confront their physicians with their anorectal problems, too often they are told that it is inadvisable to consider any surgical intervention to give local relief, since this will produce incontinence or progression of the underlying Crohn's disease.

Over the duration of the disease, the patient suffers immeasurably. In a significant percentage of cases, the rectum and anus become useless, and eventually proctocolectomy becomes necessary. It is this therapeutic nihilism that prompted us to offer surgical treatment to *selected* patients suffering from anorectal Crohn's disease. All patients in this group were suffering from undrained or incompletely drained fistulous rectal abscesses. All were symptomatic with pain. No asymptomatic fistulae were operated on.

Generally, the primary cause for fistulous abscess, in either Crohn's-related or primary fistulous disease, is the intermuscular abscess. This begins between the superficial portion of the external sphincter and the internal sphincter, the intermuscular plane. It is this plane that is the key to understanding Crohn's- or non-Crohn's–related fistulous disease, and the surgery involved. Scattered around the dentate line are 8 to 12 rectal glands. These are tubuloalveolar glands, which pierce the intermuscular plane to various extents, and, in some cases, terminate in the intermuscular plane. The posterior gland seems to be more predisposed to the development of the intermuscular abscess. Perhaps the decussation of the external sphincter renders the potential intermuscular space posteriorly more susceptible to infection. When infection has occurred within the tubuloalveolar glands, it spreads into the intermuscular plane between the sphincters to produce fistulas superficial to the external sphincter.These abscesses point on the skin surrounding the rectum or even in the scrotum or groin. In patients with Crohn's disease, the external orifice of the fistula may be located quite far from the anal verge. These types of fistulas are, of course, quite difficult to treat because of the extensive procedures needed in performing fistulotomy and fistulectomy. The procedures involve division of a significant portion of the external sphincter, rendering incontinence a distinct possibility.

If the genesis of the fistula is the intermuscular abscess, then attention to draining the abscess and removing the cryptoglandular epithelium should result in cure of the fistula without actually laying open or removing the entire fistulous track. If this basic concept is correct, the obliteration of the intermuscular abscess eventually results in healing of the fistula over a period of time. This concept was originated by Allen Parks and led to the adoption of the "Parks Procedure" or partial internal anal sphincterectomy in the treatment of Crohn's- or non-Crohn's–related fistulae.

In patients with a painful fistulous abscess, general anesthesia is used, with the patient in the lithotomy position. However, in selected cases local infiltration of the rectal area and intravenous sedation can also be used. After sigmoidoscopy to assess for associated proctitis, the Parks retractor is inserted into the rectal canal. This is a tri-blade instrument which tends to shorten the rectal canal and allow easy access to the dentate line and intermuscular space. The offending crypt where the internal orifice of the fistula is located is noted. After probing the offending gland with a crypt hook, a 1-cm strip of mucosa is removed beginning at the dentate line. This exposes the underlying internal sphincter. A fine clamp is then used to elevate a 1-cm strip of internal sphincter encompassing the rectal crypt and associated gland. This serves to drain the intermuscular space and remove the cryptoglandular epithelium. The fistulous tract is then curetted, but not removed. Occasionally, small Penrose drains are placed through the fistulous tract if it is particularly long, to achieve better drainage. It makes little difference whether the fistula is simple or complex, in the form of a bilateral horseshoe fistula. These drains are left in place for three to four days. Postoperatively, sitz baths are begun 24 hours after surgery. Antibiotics are not routinely given. Usually the patients are having frequent liquid bowel movements, and no stool softeners or laxatives are necessary or even desirable.

We believe that patients with anorectal Crohn's disease should be maintained on sulfasalazine before and after surgery. Postoperative attention to controlling the underlying Crohn's disease is emphasized. This includes prednisone, ACTH, mercaptopurine, metronidazole, and total parenteral nutrition. In particular, we are finding that mercaptopurine is useful in patients with very extensive perianal and perineal fistulae. When the patient is discharged, it is stressed that the period of time for healing of the fistula may be prolonged. Frequent office treatments are important to evaluate any further activity in the fistula. In general, the site of the sphincterectomy heals over a period of eight to sixteen weeks. The fistulous tracks, however, require a longer time to heal. Occasionally, incision and drainage along the fistulous track is necessary as an office procedure. Recurrence of an abscess in the fistulous tract will occur if the external opening of the track tends to close prior to complete obliteration of the fistulous track. Complete obliteration of the tracks usually requires four to eight months, during which time the patient is pain-free. Control of the Crohn's disease significantly increases the speed of healing of the fistulas.

We have treated 12 cases of Crohn's disease with associated painful fistulous abscesses. Healing has occurred in 11, with a median healing time, that is, sphincterectomy wound, of eight weeks. One patient required two procedures to achieve total control of recurrent abscess. While control of pain is our main criteria for success, not healing of the fistulous tracks, the fistula failed to heal in only one patient. No patient has been made incontinent by the surgery. In addition, pain has been alleviated in all cases. No patient experienced exacerbation or progression of the extrarectal Crohn's disease as a result of surgery.

The most common extrarectal site for the Crohn's disease was located in the terminal ileum and in the right colon. However, many of these patients had a combination of anorectal, ileal, and colonic Crohn's disease. While we realize that a local anorectal procedure certainly cannot prevent a high recurrence rate or the progression of extrarectal Crohn's disease, the amelioration of chronic symptoms associated with rectal disease is certainly worthwhile in selected patients. In patients with asymptomatic fistulae or those patients with perirectal discharge, treatment should be primarily medical.

The Parks procedure is a minimally invasive anorectal procedure but, in patients with partially destroyed external sphincter muscles, even removal of a portion of the internal sphincter can result in alteration of continence. In patients with severe rectal pain, drainage of the intermuscular abscess results in pain relief and, in many cases, closure of the fistula. Furthermore, this drainage prevents the continued destruction of the sphincter muscle caused by chronic abscesses. When selecting patients with anorectal Crohn's disease for anorectal surgery the full implications of the surgery must be presented to the patient. This discussion should realistically include the chances for success.

BIBLIOGRAPHY

Sohn N, Korelitz BI, Weinstein MA: Anorectal Crohn's disease, definitive surgery for fistulae and recurrent abscesses. *Am J Surg* 139:394–397, 1980.

23 An Appraisal of Surgical Procedures for Crohn's Disease

Arthur H. Aufses, Jr, MD

This chapter presents a review of the three major abdominal procedures which are done today for Crohn's disease, resection, bypass, and ileostomy or other diversionary procedures. Bypass does not refer to the operation previously discussed as bypass in continuity. We do not believe that bypass in continuity should be a procedure for Crohn's disease, although President Eisenhower had it done successfully to him. By bypass we mean bypass with exclusion of the distal side by dividing the bowel and closing the distal end.

Appraisal means: Does it work? All of these operations are successful when used for the proper indications. However, "work" does not mean cure, since we believe that every patient with Crohn's disease has Crohn's disease of his entire gastrointestinal tract. What we are concerned about is improvement of lifestyle and hope that a recurrence will not occur. If patients live long enough, they will probably all experience recurrent disease.

Resection should include the very least amount of bowel necessary to accomplish the immediate purpose. One young woman who came into the hospital in the middle of the night, fortunately many years ago, was thought to have appendicitis and taken to the operating room. Ileitis was found in the terminal ileum, and a massive resection was accomplished. This woman should not have been operated on. Once having been operated on, she should not have been resected. Once having made the decision to resect, no one today would resect the entire right colon and the midtransverse colon for this Crohn's lesion, nor would anybody remove 3 to 4 feet of normal proximal small bowel. If you happen to operate on a patient in the middle of the night and find Crohn's disease, and if the base of the cecum is normal, remove the appendix and do nothing more. If you are going to resect for Crohn's disease, go only an inch or two above the ileocecal valve if the colon is normal, saving the right colon, and go only a few inches proximal to the obvious gross extent of the disease. I personally do not have frozen sections done on the ends of the bowel. If aphthous ulcers are seen, I go a little bit further. If there is just edema of the mucosa, I am perfectly content to use that bowel. It will not leak if you do a proper anastomosis.

Resection is the preferred operation for Crohn's disease when it can be successfully accomplished. A typical case was an 18-year-old female with a string sign, multiple internal fistulae, and a large inflammatory mass. She had an ileocecal resection with an ileoascending colostomy. Her colon was spared. We went an inch or two above the ileocecal valve and took out only about four inches of the normal bowel proximal to the obvious Crohn's. A probe was left in the fistula, extending into the large mass which was in the thickened mesentery with a small abscess inside of it.

Another indication for resection is the patient who has the fistula between the ileum and sigmoid. This type of fistula is usually seen on barium enema by finding barium in the cecum and small bowel before the left colon fills. The primary disease is usually limited to the ileum. Only a small piece of the cecum and ascending colon is removed, along with a short segment of small bowel. In this case, we were unable to dissect away the ileum from the sigmoid. The inflammatory mass was too large, although the colon was intrinsically normal. A sigmoid resection, ileoascending colostomy, and a colocolostomy was done.

I would recommend that, for a patient having a double resection like this, a proximal ileostomy be done to protect both suture lines during the healing phase. I did not do it in this instance, and we were gratified that no leak occurred. If you have a patient with Crohn's disease and leave a large inflammatory area in the retroperitoneum, diversion should be performed just as you would do a transverse colostomy in a difficult patient with diverticulitis.

In general, we feel that resection is the preferred treatment. A free perforation is often considered an absolute indication for operation, but I would make a distinction. When the perforation is through the bowel wall into the free peritoneal cavity, resection must then be performed. Most of the patients with Crohn's disease who have a free perforation, however, have perforation of a mesenteric abscess, where the fistula goes from the bowel lumen into the mesentery and then out. To resect means cutting across the inflamed, infected retroperitoneal tissue. We have just drained the abscess and performed a proximal ileostomy. When the bowel wall is the site of the perforation, then obviously resection must be done. We do not make an anastomosis in the presence of diffuse peritonitis. Menguy has suggested doing a double-barreled ileocolostomy to avoid an anastomosis. We would do either an anastomosis with a proximal diversion or a double-barreled ileostomy.

In most of the patients who have had a bypass, the bowel was excluded. One patient, a 28-year-old male who had a previous bypass with exclusion, had recurrence at his ileocolostomy, with several areas of proximal disease. If this patient has to be operated on with the originally excluded loop still in place, it is believed that the excluded loop must be removed. In this situation, we remove the excluded loop, save the right colon, resect the diseased small bowel, and reestablish continuity by taking the new terminal ileum and bringing it to the ascending colon, to bring back the water-absorbing function of the ascending colon. The specimen of this patient showed that the excluded loop had become markedly fibrotic and atrophied. When the specimen is opened up, one can see that once a loop has been excluded, it fibroses very rapidly. In this case the first operation was done at the age of 21, and the second at age 28. The excluded loop is narrow, atrophic, fibrotic tissue which can never be reused. There were some patients operated on many years ago who had an exclusion, and at a subsequent operation the bowel appeared quite good. They were reanastomosed and had recurrence within days. This patient had a recurrence proximal to the anastomosis and two skip lesions.

We believe that these excluded loops should be removed. We are not doing very many bypasses with exclusions at present because of the danger of developing malignancy. In a recent review of cancer and inflammatory bowel disease, seven intestinal cancers occurred in patients with Crohn's disease with previously excluded loops. All seven were dead within two years. One cannot make a diagnosis of an excluded-loop cancer, because it is excluded and there are no symptoms. There seems to be a rather high incidence of extraintestinal cancer in these patients. If we look at these seven patients who had an excluded loop, it does not seem to make any difference whether they had the disease for a short period of time, had the exclusion, and then developed the cancer after a long period of time since the exclusion, or whether they had the disease for a long period of time, had an exclusion, and then within a short period of time developed the malignancy. The important point is that all of these patients have had ileitis or Crohn's disease in one place, whether in a functioning segment or not, for many years. As a consequence, we believe that you have the same problem here that you do in ulcerative colitis: long-standing disease in place is a cancer risk. The risk is not as high as in ulcerative colitis. It is probably less than half that risk, but it is a risk nevertheless.

Finally, let us consider the use of ileostomy as a staging procedure in Crohn's disease and provide some examples where a preliminary ileostomy is preferable. One example was a patient with an ileosigmoid fistula, a large inflammatory mass, temperature of 102°F, involvement of the bladder without a vesical fistula and, at operation, involvement of the retroperitoneum by the inflammatory mass and abscess. Only a proximal ileostomy was done. The mass disappeared within a month. After three to four months, the now more localized disease was resected. An ileoascending colostomy was done, the fistula was closed, and the ileostomy was left in place. At a later date, when it was certain that both suture lines were healed, the ileostomy was closed.

Other situations where we have done this have been in patients with a perforation of a mesenteric abscess. One patient with ileitis and a large mesenteric abscess developed diffuse peritonitis from rupture of the abscess. The abscess was drained through the flank and a proximal ileostomy was done. Subsequently, this patient had a resection and the ileostomy was closed. If the rectum was normal at the time we did the ileostomy; every patient subsequently had intestinal continuity restored and was able to use the rectum.

Another example was a patient with a large retroperitoneal abscess which caused a hydronephrosis. This particular individual presented with the abscess pointing at the back as a psoas abscess, and the abscess was drained through the back. An ileostomy was then done. When she had the bowel resection performed a year later, her kidney and ureter had completely returned to normal. Our experience has been that one never has to operate on the kidney or ureter specifically in patients with Crohn's disease. If the retroperitoneal infection and bowel are managed, the kidney and the ureter take care of themselves.

A similar situation was a young woman with extensive ileocolitis and fistulae, a mesenteric abscess in the sigmoid, and hydronephrosis on the left side. The only procedure that was done was drainage of the abscess and ileostomy. Subsequently, she had a staged proctocolectomy. She has had other troubles, but is now essentially well. When she had the ileostomy, we knew she could never use her rectum again because of extensive rectal disease.

Finally, a patient with an ileosigmoid anastomosis was operated on for acute intestinal obstruction, after not responding to long tube and having an unprepared distended bowel. Only an ileostomy was done as a preliminary procedure. Subsequently, she went on to have a resection and reestablishment of continuity.

PANEL DISCUSSION

Question: I would like Dr Korelitz to comment further on the figures for recurrence rates after ileostomy.

Dr Korelitz: I was comparing them with the figure from my earlier study at Mt Sinai Hospital, which was 46% after many different periods of follow-up. Others had reported anywhere from 0% to 33%. My figure was high, but now other institutions are reporting similar figures.

Question: What is the best management for rectovaginal fistula?

Dr Weinstein: The group that we presented did not include rectovaginal fistula. If the fistula is symptomatic, with pain, and there is an associated intermuscular abscess, the abscess should be drained. However, one must inform the patient that the fistula may become more active. A direct attack on the fistula itself is doomed to failure. Some of these patients with large fistulas do become candidates for proctocolectomy. If there is an associated abscess with the fistula, then you can help them a little bit.

Dr Korelitz: Many rectovaginal fistulae dry up with mercaptopurine. The potential space remains, air might still come through, but the fistula stops draining and the patient is perfectly comfortable.

Dr Aufses: I would like to ask Dr Korelitz: About recurrences in patients who had stomas, three of which subsequently had a radical procedure for neoplasm. What were those three neoplasms?

Dr Korelitz: One was a melanoma, one a hypernephroma, and the third, a breast carcinoma.

Dr Steichen: You showed a very interesting case in which the patient presented with an abscess. You performed first a proximal diversion and then you reoperated. Would there be an alternate approach? For instance, if the patient were quite sick, undernourished, and presented with an abscess, would you continue hyperalimentation, perhaps drain the abscess, but not do the diversion? What is your experience in the use of hyperalimentation in such a patient.

Dr Sohn: I think that particular patient was operated upon before we had hyperalimentation. You are absolutely right that today one could make a case for trying to treat the patient either with simple drainage of the abscess and hyperalimentation, or hyperalimentation alone. I have seen large masses get much smaller or even disappear. We have not been able to reproduce Dudrick's successes with long-term hyperalimentation, but I suspect it is because we have not given it for as long a period of time. We are not very anxious to keep patients in the hospital for three to four months on hyperalimentation, and we do not have a home hyperalimentation program developed to the extent that they have in Texas. It can certainly help tide you over a difficult situation. I would suspect that today most of our ileostomies are being done in a true emergency situation. That patient with the large abscess was an electively scheduled operation.

Dr Steichen: What is your opinion as to when to use hyperalimentation in a patient with a fistula, an abscess plus fistula to the abdominal wall, or a fistula to another organ, where previous operations have been performed and you are not too eager to intervene again? There are a large number of patients with indolent, chronic problems, and in the past we really did not have too much to offer them. We now can improve alimentation and may heal the fistulae. What is the experience of the various members of the panel?

Dr Sohn: The ASPEN (American Society of Parenteral and Enteral Nutrition) group had certain criteria for hyperalimentation which probably applies to Crohn's and other diseases. Such patients may have a serum albumin of less than 3.4 mg/dl. If the patient is anergic or if there is a weight loss of 10 lbs, that patient becomes a candidate for nutritional support. In these patients, we are really talking about using a central modality because the protein-sparing and the peripheral TPN that Dr Robbins spoke about do not seem to reverse the metabolism in these very sick patients.

Dr Weinstein: When we are dealing with any patient who is sick with inflammatory bowel disease, we generally start them on hyperalimentation, usually within the first 48 hours. We consider it part of the therapy for severe, acute disease and feel that it may help the patient avoid an operation. If the patient does respond to the medical therapy and should come to surgery, he would be in a more optimal physiologic state.

Dr Korelitz: Hyperalimentation buys time. Therefore, it must be included with something else as part of a dual plan. One can anticipate improvement with the hyperalimentation, but what are you going to do once that improvement has been accomplished?

Dr Steichen: In other words, we try to improve the patient's general condition by hyperalimentation, antibiotics, etc. This is never really a treatment per se.

Dr Korelitz: This is based on the presumption that after you stop it, the original clinical situation will recur, slowly or quickly.

Dr Sohn: Dudrick has reported long-term successful amelioration of symptoms. We have not been able to reproduce that. My own indication for hyperalimentation is what has just been alluded to: the bad risk patient who is hospitalized to buy some time. We recently had a young man with an enterocutaneous fistula. We put him on hyperalimentation and the fistula was closed within four to five days, and the mass almost disappeared. We continued the hyperalimentation for three weeks. He was perfectly well. We stopped the hyperalimintation and put him back on diet. Within a week the mass was back, and before he left the hospital we had to do a resection. I have not seen a long-term good result with a patient remaining well by the use of hyperalimentation as the only mode of therapy. These patients require something else, either medical management or a subsequent surgical procedure.

Dr Sohn: One situation where TPN is more than adjunctive therapy and probably is the definitive modality (despite the fact that you are using other medical modalities) is in cases of fistulae, particularly postoperative fistulae, which may have nothing to do with the Crohn's disease per se. These fistulae can be closed, using TPN. I think the TPN is important here. Dr Robbins presented one case this morning where the patient had four to five weeks of TPN, had an abscess drained with a resultant enterocutaneous fistula. He was treated with mercaptopurine or sulfasalazine and steroids, but this was a patient where I felt the TPN was more important than the other forms of therapy.

Question: In Crohn's disease, if a patient has had a resection with removal of the grossly apparent disease, and he is asymptomatic, should he be kept on sulfasalazine and at what dosage?

Dr Korelitz: The studies that would answer this have not yet been completed. I have used sulfasalazine beginning in the postoperative period, in the hope that eventually it might have some prophylactic value. In some patients whose courses have been particularly virulent up until that point and have already had two to three resections, I would use mercaptopurine prophylactically.

Dr Aufses: I would not argue with the use of sulfasalazine postoperatively, since it probably could not do any harm, but I believe that it is going to take a long time before one of those studies gives a definitive answer. One of Crohn's patients reported in 1932 came back to Mount Sinai Hospital in 1965, 33 years later, with a recurrence that had just become symptomatic. It is going to take many studies, over a long period of time, to obtain the answer.

Question: I am wondering why several groups in Boston have lower postoperative recurrence rates in Crohn's disease.

Dr Korelitz: I have wondered that for a long time myself. Perhaps it is a different disease in New England.

Dr Steichen: One last question about the patient who comes back a second or third time with recurrence after surgery, appears to be a very clear indication for the operation. But now the patient has already lost small bowel and is about to lose more. One then approaches the problem differently.

Dr Korelitz: First, I hope I do not give the impression that I am against surgery. The problem is that Crohn's disease is relentless. Somebody has to put the brake on somewhere, and postpone surgery for the right time. The right time might prove to be never. Admittedly the "right" time is an area of controversy. Usually the nature of the recurrence is the same as the nature of the original disease. It is often clear in retrospect that the patient might have gotten by without having been operated on the first time, but then it is too late to do anything. So, if I had not had the option of stopping it earlier, I would make every effort to stop it now, and give the patient all medical options.

Dr Steichen: I would use the word nonoperative. For most of you, there are two treatments: medical and surgical. As a surgeon, there are also two treatments: operative and nonoperative. The possibility of a recurrence always exists. When the surgeon makes the decision to operate for the first time, he must contemplate the possibility of a recurrence and what he will do when this happens. If there is an area of narrowing that is causing an obstruction, for instance, that area should be resected. Basically, we are not going to cure the disease with any operation; the procedure should be designed to improve the patient's physiologic status.

Dr Aufses: I would agree, but I think we will all think a bit longer and a bit more about the patient who has had multiple small bowel resections.

For almost 20 years, I have been measuring the amount of small bowel in every patient I operate on for Crohn's disease. I was impressed with the fact that a large number of these patients seem to have much less small bowel than the patient operated on for carcinoma. It was one of the things that led me to believe many years ago that Crohn's disease was one involving the whole bowel, even though you could not see it. I have continued to measure the amount of small bowel on every patient. I think that if you can leave a patient with 5 or 6 feet of small bowel attached to normal colon, that is the key. Whatever colon you are using has to be normal, even if it is only the rectum. If you can have 5 or 6 feet of apparently normal small bowel and a normal section piece of colon, that patient will not be an intestinal "cripple." He will never become robust, but will survive on diet adjustments.

We have some patients on supplemental home hyperalimentation. They have a fistula or a Scribner shunt inserted. They are able to give themselves the home hyperalimentation, but have to return to the hospital to get it started.

24 What is the Best Medical Management for Ulcerative Colitis?

Richard G. Farmer, MD

Studies have recently shown that for a hospital-based gastroenterologist, the largest single disease state now seen is inflammatory bowel disease (IBD). Thus, the problem of IBD is a very significant one, particularly so for those who are primarily concerned with digestive disease. Furthermore, in an attempt to define what services internists and subspecialists provide, various terminologies have been developed for statistical and data collecting purposes. The terms primary care, secondary care, tertiary care, and principal care have been defined by medical planners. Principal care includes the patient with a chronic disease for whom the patient's major care is handled by a specialist, either an internist or subspecialist. In terms of principal care patients, IBD ranks at the top of the list for gastroenterologists.

In hearings before the National Commission on Digestive Disease, it became apparent that one of the major problems encountered in IBD from the patient's point of view, is a sense of isolation, loneliness, and derision because of the disease. Many physicians, especially house officers, have a sterotyped picture of the patient with IBD. Thus, the first point in managing such a patient is rapport. Appropriate rapport includes an understanding that the patient feels a sense of derision, a sense of loneliness, and a sense that nobody wants to talk about his disease. A patient who has recovered from cancer, heart surgery, or other major diseases often has a kind of heroic attitude. However, the patient who is improved but not cured of a disease causing fistulas, diarrhea, and malnutrition often does not have the feeling of heroism or support from others. This can be a very important consideration in patient management.

The second point is that IBD has become relatively common. In our gastrointestinal unit last year we saw over 1500 patients with IBD. A major problem in their management is the relative unpredictability of various modalities of treatment, as evidenced by the wide range of response to the same program in a large population.

The goal in treating these patients is to have them function as normally as possible, and to allow them a reasonably normal diet. Often, the value of diet, rest, graded exercise, and other activities are not emphasized as much as in the past. Nevertheless, it is important to try to get the patient functioning as nearly normally as possible under their circumstances of physical strength, nutrition and systems. If a person is 25 lbs underweight and has a fistula and synovitis, he is not going to be very active physically, and his diet will be restricted because of malaise and anorexia. A high protein diet is, of course, valuable. Once the patient leaves the hospital, physical and other activities become very important. This is particularly true for the adolescent patient. Although much has been written about the prepubertal patient or the one with hyperalimentation and short bowel syndrome, these do not represent large numbers of patients with IBD. A very common type of patient is the late teenager who is not growth-retarded, but is chronically ill. This is at a time in their lives when they are trying to be economically and psychologically independent, and their disease has rendered them just the opposite. Often, the response of their parents and families is to exaggerate this. Many of the psychological problems of IBD relate to this phenomenon. An understanding physician who provides principal care represents an important service to the patient, and this type of understanding can be significant in management.

With regard to medications, I recommend the use of supportive therapy for symptoms, but no more than is necessary. I do not recommend, for example, putting *all* patients on an antispasmodic, an antidiarrheal, a tranquilizer, a pain medication, plus an antiinflammatory agent, unless this seems to be absolutely necessary.

In terms of what type of "specific" medication should be used, sulfasalazine has been available since the 1940s, although its exact mechanism of action is still poorly understood. It is known that sulfasalazine is decomposed by colonic bacteria into 5-ASA (salicylate) and sulfapyridine, and its primary effect appears to be on the ileum and colon. Its use on a short-term basis to control symptoms, flare ups of disease, and the disease itself, is well established, and long-term use is also advocated. However, there are conflicting studies as to the efficacy of long-term use of sulfasalazine on either a prophylactic basis or for recurrences. Use in ulcerative colitis has been studied more extensively than in Crohn's disease. The fact that sulfasalazine was used for about 20 years before randomized, double-blind, prospective studies were done, has led to difficulty in assessing its efficacy. However, the disease itself has caused problems in evaluating the results. Nevertheless, in ulcerative colitis, in contrast to Crohn's disease, the most frequently used therapy is sulfasalazine. Prednisone has also been used extensively in treatment of ulcerative colitis, which can be identical to the treatment of Crohn's disease. A common program is the relatively short-term use of steroid in conjunction with sulfasalazine, with subsequent tapering of the dose of prednisone.

In summary, as far as drug therapy is concerned, I favor sulfasalazine, in a dose of 2 to 4 grams, on a fairly long-term basis for ulcerative colitis. One should recognize that this is empirical therapy, and criteria for improvement must be established. The use of prednisone intermittently for a relatively short period of time may supplement sulfasalazine. The use of immunosuppressives in ulcerative colitis is not as well recognized as in Crohn's disease, because of the relatively better response by patients with ulcerative colitis than those with Crohn's disease, plus the long-term concern about the development of cancer.

In drug treatment there are four factors which relate to the patient's therapeutic response. The first is the age of the patient. The second is the clinical severity of the disease as well as its extent. The third is the duration of the illness and the fourth is the family, social, personal, and work situation. All four of these factors may alter the apparent response to either sulfasalazine or prednisone, and often in a somewhat unpredictable manner. Patients who have had the disease for a long time, and have already been treated with other medications, have a different set of problems and complications than the patient in the initial stage of the disease. Likewise, the age of the patient, whether prepubertal, postpubertal, or adult, and the severity of the disease, alter the response. There are some patients in whom the disease is inexorably progressive, usually in a rather acute phase, where response to therapy is poor. Thus, it is possible to incorrectly attribute response or lack of it under various circumstances.

There are basically four indications for surgery in ulcerative colitis: toxic megacolon, acute hemorrhage, chronic illness with debility, and concern over cancer. The most frequent of these is chronic debility.

In ulcerative colitis, in contrast with Crohn's disease, there may be two alternatives to a permanent ileostomy, an ileorectal anastomosis and a Kock pouch. With ileorectal anastomosis it is possible that cancer will develop in the remaining rectal segment. Both of these operations are relatively uncommon. Most patients require a standard ileostomy. A cancer surveillance program in ulcerative colitis is very important. Finally, I would emphasize the use of consultants: the surgeon, the nutritionist, and the psychiatrist. The "team" approach is important, but the principal care must still be maintained by the internist or gastroenterologist.

We have studied 371 patients with ulcerative proctosigmoiditis, with a 97% 11-year follow-up, and have found, that 90% have a good prognosis. We have treated these patients primarily with hydrocortisone enemas as the sole form of therapy, using a three-week course, stopping for a week, and repeating the course if necessary. We attempt to avoid systemic medication if possible, but use sulfasalazine if necessary.

An example of long-term follow-up of patients with ulcerative colitis is our group of children and teenagers. There were 316 patients in this study, with a follow-up of ten years and about a 5% mortality rate. Only one third were operated on, which is a very important point because of the long-term potential for cancer. The most common complication was what can be called chronic disease with diarrhea, rectal bleeding, and weight loss over a protracted period. Ten of the patients had toxic megacolon and seven had growth retardation. The most important statistic is that the patients seen from 1955 to 1965, compared with those seen from 1965 to 1975, had approximately twice the number of operations. One could say the disease has become less severe, that our philosophy about surgery has changed, or that the treatment is better. In our experience, most operations take place within the first five years after onset of the disease. Thus, there are now a large number of patients — over 200 who were teenagers at the time of onset of ulcerative colitis – who have now been followed for ten years, and therefore are at risk of developing colonic cancer. Many of these are relatively asymptomatic. They may have changed physicians, may have moved away, and often may not be particularly interested in undergoing an elaborate surveillance program. This is one of the major problems in the treatment of ulcerative colitis, ie, a rational surveillance program and patient compliance.

Finally, what is the quality of life for a patient who has had ulcerative colitis for more than ten years? For most patients it is not bad, but studies have shown that one-half to two-thirds of our patients are functioning in what they would regard as a suboptimal manner. Even though their symptoms may have improved, and even though they may not have had an operation, most patients do not feel that their health is as good as their contemporaries'. The attitude of "chronic illness" can be a significant factor.

The physician must maintain objectivity regarding the principal care, consultations, the family, and the nutritional state of the patient, and must react in an objective manner to the various problems. Concern over the patient's welfare and a sensitivity toward the patient are quite important. However, the physician must be very careful to maintain objectivity, particularly about the decision leading to colectomy and ileostomy.

25 Why Do Results of Management of Toxic Megacolon Differ?

Michael J. Schmerin, MD

Toxic megacolon or toxic dilatation of the colon is an ominous complication of inflammatory bowel disease (IBD). It is characterized by acute dilatation of the colon to greater than six cm in diameter and is associated with signs of systemic toxicity. Classically, toxic megacolon is associated with the fulminant phase of ulcerative colitis, but it has also been described in other disease states and is a recognized complication of granulomatous or Crohn's colitis as well. It has been described in patients with pseudomembranous colitis secondary to antibiotic usage, ischemic colitis, and infectious colitis secondary to shigellosis or amebiasis.

The incidence of toxic megacolon varies from 1.6% to 6% of patients with ulcerative colitis. Most episodes develop during a relapse of chronic ulcerative colitis, yet approximately 25% to 33% of the attacks occur during the acute initial episode. The actual cause of the dilatation is not known. In a small group of patients reported two years ago, cytomegalovirus was recovered from the colon of patients with toxic megacolon. Other attempts to isolate specific infectious or toxic agents have been unsuccessful to date. Pathologically, there is severe transmural destruction of the circular and longitudinal muscles of the colon, as well as acute inflammatory changes extending through the wall to the serosa. The destruction is most severe in the dilated sections of the colon, but there is inflammation throughout for the most part. There was also evidence of vasculitis occurring as well as inflammation of the myenteric nerve plexuses, but these findings were variable and probably not responsible for the syndrome. In fact, at this point, no unique inflammatory change has been found to account for toxic megacolon. When one examines the gross specimen that has been removed surgically, severe extensive ulcerations are found. In some specimens, more than 50% of the mucosa can be destroyed. In the areas of extensive ulceration, the bowel is extremely friable and thin. In fact, it resembles wet tissue paper and is often no more than 2 mm to 3 mm thick.

Important in any patient with toxic megacolon are the possible precipitating factors in the development of the toxic dilatation. These factors promote high intraluminal pressure or decreased colonic muscle tone. Precipitating factors which have been identified include opiates, anticholinergics, the administration of a barium enema prior to the development of toxic megacolon, colonoscopy in a few cases prior to the development of toxic megacolon, hypokalemia, and rapidly progressive disease. Norland and Kirsner found that 64% of their cases were precipitated by one of the above-mentioned factors, while Hartong and his associates at the University of Kansas found that 70% of their cases were anteceded by either drugs or a barium enema. In Norland's study of patients who were given narcotics, 50% had received them for less than 48 hours before the onset of toxic megacolon. In another series, 94% of patients had been on anticholinergics from days to months before the onset of the toxic megacolon. It has been the impression of numerous clinicians that in fulminant colitis, the colon is more sensitive to anticholinergics and opiates, and that dilatation is more readily induced with even smaller doses of the drug than usual. Of course, this is a clinical observation and has not been proven in the laboratory.

What is the clinical picture of the patient with toxic megacolon? Essentially it is that of a severely ill patient. The patient has tachycardia of 100 to 140 beats per minute, fever as high as 104°F, dehydration, and abdominal pain. However, the abdominal pain is not necessarily localized to any one particular quadrant. It can be generalized. Physical examination is remarkable, primarily for diminished to absent bowel sounds, tympany, and mild rebound tenderness. The lungs are clear and cardiac examination reveals the tachycardia. Laboratory evaluation is basically nonspecific. There is commonly leukocytosis and anemia (presumably secondary to iron deficiency), hypoalbuminemia, and an elevated sedimentation rate. The diagnosis is made from the abdominal flat film. There we see dilatation of all or part of the colon to more than 6 cm. Classically, it is in the transverse colon. This confirms the diagnosis. Also found on the flat and upright films is the irregular serrated colonic mucosa, which sometimes can be outlined. One may also see small bowel distention, but gastric dilatation is unusual. Very important to look for on the flat plate is free air under the diaphragm, which suggests a perforated colon, a common complication of toxic dilatation.

The treatment of toxic megacolon can be divided into three groups: general medical treatment to support the patient, specific medical treatment aimed at treating the colitis, and surgical treatment.

The medical treatment of toxic megacolon is intensive. Its value is still being debated in the medical and surgical literature. There are those who feel that medical therapy has a minimal role, and that the patient should be operated on as a surgical emergency. There are also those who wait and treat medically, often suboptimally and for too long a period. At Lenox Hill Hospital, we treat toxic megacolon as an aggressive medical disease. General medical therapy includes intravenous fluid replacement, sufficient to make up for the losses due to dehydration. This may require 4 to 5 liters per day. Electrolyte abnormalities should be corrected vigorously, especially hypokalemia, which may play a precipitating role in the toxic megacolon. We place a small bowel tube for constant suction. Salt-poor albumin is replaced to bring the albumin level up to normal. Blood transfusions are necessary to increase the hematocrit to a range of 33 to 36. In certain cases a rectal tube can be used to aid in decompression of the colon. All opiates and anticholinergics, which the patient may have been taking, are discontinued. The patient is placed at complete bowel rest, and broad-spectrum antibiotics are given intravenously. Various combinations have been used such as cefazolin and gentamycin or ampicillin, clindamycin and gentamycin, or chloramphenicol and gentamycin. I favor the latter two combinations, because this includes anaerobic coverage as well.

The role of steroids in the treatment of toxic megacolon is still questionable. In a recent issue of *Gastroenterology,* Myers and co-workers evaluated the evidence to date for the use of steroids in toxic megacolon. They could not determine if steroids favorably affect the outcome of toxic dilatation. They did note, however, that steroids do not appear to worsen the outcome. We believe that steroids have had a favorable influence and should be used. High doses of ACTH, 60 to 80 units every eight hours intravenously are used. Other clinicians prefer intravenous prednisone or hydrocortisone with possibly equal results. Our clinical experience suggests that ACTH is superior to prednisone or hydrocortisone. However, a satisfactory controlled study has not been done. It is also important to remember that by the time one sees patients with toxic megacolon, most will have been on steroids for treatment of their underlying disease. Therefore, they will require increased doses in order to prevent relative adrenal insufficiency in view of the new stress they are undergoing. The patient often must be monitored carefully in an intensive care setting. Toxic megacolon is a medical emergency, and the patient should be evaluated every four to six hours. The abdominal girth should be measured for clinical appraisal, and daily flat films obtained and reviewed. If response is not apparent by clinical examination by radiographic evidence of decreased dilatation, surgery should be considered after 72 hours.

Of course, there are specific indications for surgery, the most important being perforation. Next is impending perforation. Another is a deteriorating clinical course after 72 hours on a maximal medical regimen such as described above. Severe hemorrhage, though unusual, is an indication for surgery. The last indication is persistent colonic dilatation beyond one week, but that is less well defined than the others. There have been cases of patients who are relatively asymptomatic and have a persistent dilatation on flat plate. Therefore, the decision to operate for persistent colonic dilatation must be based on the clinical status of the patient.

The most common and serious complication is free perforation of the colon. Even if surgery is performed immediately for suspected perforation, a review of the literature reveals the mortality rate to be as high as 50%.

Complications other than perforation of toxic megacolon include gram-negative bacteremia and sepsis. We are trying to prevent this initially with antibiotic therapy. Thrombophlebitis and pulmonary emboli also can occur, especially in the patient who is at bedrest. Of course, it is very difficult to advocate anticoagulation in the patient who may develop one of the other complications such as massive rectal hemorrhage. Acute tubular necrosis has been reported, and this may possibly be prevented by vigorous fluid replacement.

A recent review by Binder et al concerned 497 patients with toxic megacolon, and showed that approximately 30% were successfully managed medically. There was an overall mortality rate in the medically treated patients of 30% and surgery was required in the other 40%.

What are the statistics for the surgical operation? Surgical mortality in toxic megacolon without perforation is approximately 8% to 10% but, if perforation has occurred, it rises to approximately 50%. Since perforation is the most incriminating factor in the high mortality rate associated with toxic megacolon, the keystone to successful management is avoidance of colonic perforation. It seems that neither the previous duration of colitis nor the magnitude of the dilatation, are related to the final outcome in terms of perforation. If surgery is necessary, a total proctocolectomy with ileostomy is the procedure of choice. In some instances, depending on the judgment of the surgeon, if the patient is desperately ill, a subtotal colectomy leaving the rectal stump may be favored with justification. Less definitive procedures are only temporizing compromises and further surgery will usually be required.

In summary, toxic megacolon with or without perforation is a severe complication of IBD. It requires prompt and intensive medical care, and it is important to realize that a significant number of patients will require surgery.

BIBLIOGRAPHY

Binder SC, Patterson JF, Glotzer DJ: Toxic megacolon in ulcerative colitis. *Gastroenterology* 66:909–915, 1974.

Hartong WA, Arvantahis C, Skibba RM, et al: Treatment of toxic megacolon. *Digestive Diseases* 22:195–200, 1977.

Koudahl G, Kristensen M: Toxic megacolon in ulcerative colitis. *Scand J Gastroenterol* 10:417–421, 1975.

Marshak RH, Korelitz BI, Klein SH, et al: Toxic dilation of the colon in the course of ulcerative colitis. *Gastroenterology* 38:165–180, 1960.

Meyers S, Janowitz HD: The place of steroids in the therapy of toxic megacolon. *Gastroenterology* 75:729–731, 1978.

Norland CC, Kirsner JB: Toxic dilation of the colon: etiology, treatment, and prognosis in 42 patients. *Medicine* 48:229–250, 1969.

Ripstein CB, Weiner ED: Toxic megacolon. *Dis Colon Rectum* 16:402–408, 1973.

Scott WH, Sawyer JL, Gobbel WG, et al: Surgical management of toxic dilation of the colon in ulcerative colitis. *Ann Surg* 179:647–656, 1974.

Smith FW, Law DH, Nichel WF, et al: Fulminant ulcerative colitis with toxic dilation of the colon. *Gastroenterology* 42:233–243, 1962.

26 An Appraisal of the Cancer Problem in Ulcerative Colitis

Richard G. Farmer, MD

The problem of cancer in ulcerative colitis is a very important one, although not so important numerically as it is emotionally. We encounter approximately four cancers in ulcerative colitis per year. There is a group of at least 200 ex-teenagers whom we have followed for ten years, who still have their colons and are at high risk for colonic cancer. For effective surveillance for cancer, there must be a system which is cost-effective and ensure patient compliance. The patient may be frightened of the cancer risk and feel there is a "sword hanging over his head" for the rest of his life. He may feel that because he has ulcerative colitis, sooner or later he is going to have to have a colectomy. However, some type of rational approach is important.

What patient is at highest risk of getting cancer? There are really only two factors that have stood the test of time. The first is a duration of colitis over ten years, and the second is the extent of the colitis involving the entire colon. All other factors have not proven to be statistically significant in terms of being predictable risk factors for subsequent development of cancer. These factors include less than total colon involvement, activity of disease, quiescence of disease, severity of onset, number of episodes, use of steroids, and extracolonic manifestations. This leaves us with a poor ability to anticipate which patient might get cancer. Therefore an extremely valuable modality has been the use of endoscopy.

We have been studying the use of colonoscopy in inflammatory bowel disease (IBD) for the past five years, and have attempted to define "diagnostic" colonoscopy and "surveillance" colonoscopy in ulcerative colitis. We have also attempted to define dysplasia, which is not well defined histologically. This problem led the National Foundation for Ileitis and Colitis to sponsor a national meeting on the subject of dysplasia, from which a better understanding has developed.

We define diagnostic colonoscopy as colonoscopy which has been performed for some diagnostic purpose, such as radiographic, abnormality, the determination of disease activity, differential diagnosis between Crohn's disease and ulcerative colitis, or another specific reason. Surveillance colonoscopy, on the other hand, is indicated in a patient who has had ten years of ulcerative colitis and total colon disease, for whom we are trying to determine whether or not there is a potential for cancer or whether or not dysplasia exists. We studied 89 cases of colonoscopy, 49 surveillance and 40 diagnostic. We also attempted to define what dysplasia means. We believe that abnormalities in the nuclei and increased mitotic activity in association with relatively atrophic mucosa and only minimal inflammation are the most significant findings. One cannot assess dysplasia in the presence of very active disease, because of regenerative changes.

In the 40 diagnostic colonoscopies, seven patients were found to have dysplasia and five of them were found to have cancer. Of the patients who did not have dysplasia, none had cancer. There were three cancers found in the diagnostic survey, and all three also had dysplasia close to or distal from the lesion.

Thus, as far as the diagnostic colonoscopy is concerned, five of the seven patients with dysplasia proved to have cancer. No patients without dysplasia had cancer, and all three cancer patients had dysplasia. For surveillance colonoscopy, eight patients were found to have dysplasia; two of the eight had cancer. No dysplasia was present in 38, and no cancers were found. However, two cancers and one tubulovillous adenoma were found incidentally. There was a correlation of no dysplasia — no cancer in this group of patients. Those patients who were operated on for other reasons and who had no dysplasia, did not have cancer. Of those patients who did have dysplasia, five of the seven had cancer. Thus, there were 11 cancers found in these 75 patients over this five-year period. Of the patients without an operation, two have had more biopsies; one still had dysplasia. There was no subsequent biopsy in six of these patients.

When the indication for endoscopy was for surveillance, four of 49 patients had cancer. This was found on endoscopy, and the colonoscopy was performed because the patient had ten years of ulcerative colitis. With regard to duration of disease, among patients with less than ten years' duration, three patients had dysplasia and 12 patients whose duration of disease was over ten years had dysplasia. Thus there is a correlation between duration of disease, presence of dysplasia, and presence of cancer. We are seeing much more quiescent disease, in that 9 of the 11 cancers were in patients with quiescent disease.

There were two patients in whom the cancer was grossly unrecognized. The lesion was submucosal, multifocal, superficial, and spreading. Histologic specimens of all patients were sent to five pathologists in a blind way at sporadic intervals. They agreed 92% of the time. This is significant.

Therefore, we have found that dysplasia is present in patients who have colonic cancer with ulcerative colitis, and that all the patients who have cancer have dysplasia.

However, not all patients who had dysplasia had cancer. We believe that colonoscopy with multiple biopsies is a valuable technique, and at the present time are recommending colonoscopy with multiple biopsies every one to two years for patients with ulcerative colitis of greater than ten years' duration.

There is now a reasonably large number of patients with ulcerative colitis of ten or more years' duration who are at higher risk for developing colonic cancer than the general population. Thus, there is need to have surveillance programs for cancer which are both effective and cost-effective, and which insure as much compliance from the patient as possible.

27 The Problems Arising in Diagnosis of Dysplasia as a Premalignant Lesion in Ulcerative Colitis

Sheldon C. Sommers, MD*

Dysplasia in the uterine cervix and in the skin has criteria which are generally recognized and uniform throughout the country. In the case of the uterine cervix, carcinoma in situ and dysplasia of various grades became a subject of interest about 1945. For the next ten years, it was uncertain what the borderlines of the histologic diagnosis of any of these were, until uniform criteria were established. There are other places in the body, such as the breast epithelium and the endometrium, where exact criteria for different degrees of dysplasia and carcinoma in situ are still in question. For the endometrium, the argument has been going on for 80 years. There are other epithelia, like those of the pancreatic ducts and the prostate, where uniform criteria do not exist. In the colon, the situation is somewhat like that of the uterine cervix between 1945 and 1955. Dysplasia in the colon exists, and it is possible to recognize it, but the means for grading it requires further work.

Cancer of the large bowel may be the most common internal human cancer. Because less than 1% of the cases of complicating ulcerative colitis make up large bowel carcinomas, it is important to recognize these cases as carcinomas. For example, the

---

*With the assistance of Charlotte Moss Fox.

literature reports that if dysplasia of the colon is found on biopsy, and a colectomy is done, cancer will be found in 40% of the cases. That has not been our experience. In Dr Korelitz's material of over 500 sigmoidoscopic biopsies, there was significant dysplasia in 12 cases. Of these 12, only one had a colectomy. That was a child with severe dysplasia, and no cancer was found. This indicates a marked discrepancy between our experience and that reported in the literature.

Pseudopolyps in ulcerative colitis are persistent, inflamed areas of mucosa, overhanging ulcers. They are in no way precancerous. In fact, histologically, pseudopolyps are largely granulation tissue. Although the epithelium may look disturbed, it almost never shows real dysplasia. Today no one believes that carcinomas arise in pseudopolyps.

Table 27-1 illustrates the differences between carcinoma of the colon with and without predisposing ulcerative colitis.

Table 27-1
Differences Between Carcinoma of Colon
With and Without Predisposing Ulcerative Colitis

	No UC	UC
Ratio of frequency	1	10–20
Lesion identified by radiologist	99%	70%
Overhanging edges by x-ray	***	*
Stricture by x-ray	*	***
Recognition as carcinoma by radiologist	95%	40%

The radiologist can recognize only about 70% of the lesions. The tumors do not have the typical napkin-ring or cauliflower appearance by x-ray. Stricture is often a site where carcinoma arises in ulcerative colitis. The radiologist finds somewhat less than 40% of cases as diagnosable large bowel carcinomas.

The involvement of the entire colon together with a disease duration of ten years or more are important, particularly if the onset is in childhood. It has been reported, however, that 22% of carcinomas arising in ulcerative colitis developed before ten years of activity had elapsed.

From the viewpoint of the pathologist, there are five distinctive features of carcinoma in ulcerative colitis:

1. Unusually undifferentiated carcinomas, which are not seen in people without ulcerative colitis.
2. In some cases development of other types of tumors, such as Hodgkin's disease, as a complication of ulcerative colitis. The combined clinical and pathologic accuracy before microscopic examination is somewhat under 65%.
3. Multiple synchronous or asynchronous separate primary carcinomas.
4. Occurrence in younger age groups than in those not having ulcerative colitis.
5. Uniform distribution of the cancers throughout the whole colon.

Riddell has reported, however, that 40% of carcinomas accompanying ulcerative colitis are in the rectosigmoid or rectum, and that only 60% are above that. More often they are mucinous carcinomas.

Dysplasia develops in other parts of the colon of the individual who has carcinoma with ulcerative colitis. In inflamed, active degeneration, ulceration and regeneration, one must disregard the hyperchromatism, the palisading, and the irregularity of some of the crypts. The same applies to the recognition of dysplasia in the chronically inflamed gastric mucosa and in chronic endometritis. In both places, very atypical epithelium is downgraded to no dysplasia, if there is inflammation present. Apparently this is an epithelial change secondary to inflammation and not independent epithelial activity.

Figures 27-1 and 27-2 show what was originally thought to be severe dysplasia in a very inflamed environment. The cells are acidophilic in the crypt. They are very irregular in their nuclear size and arrangement, both in the crypt and on the surface. However, after consultation it was decided that this was metaplasia, and not a significant or real dysplasia. Subsequent biopsies on this patient showed no dysplasia; she still has her colon.

Figure 27-3 illustrates a biopsy from another patient. All three pathologists consulted at first thought these must be carcinoma cells. Then, noting the degree of inflammation intimately mixed with the epithelial cells, the lesion was diagnosed as a pseudodysplasia or pseudocarcinoma. Subsequent biopsies have not shown any dysplasia, and this patient kept his colon as well.

One of the specimens of ulcerative colitis has a villous hyperplasia, and under high power the most important area is down near the bases of the crypts (Figure 27-4). Since there is active inflammation, the degree of atypia is probably not significant (Figure 27-5). In some crypts of these cases with villous hyperplasia, there is very little irregularity of the epithelium, either in arrangement or nuclear size. Table 27-2 lists the historic criteria that are useful for the pathologist.

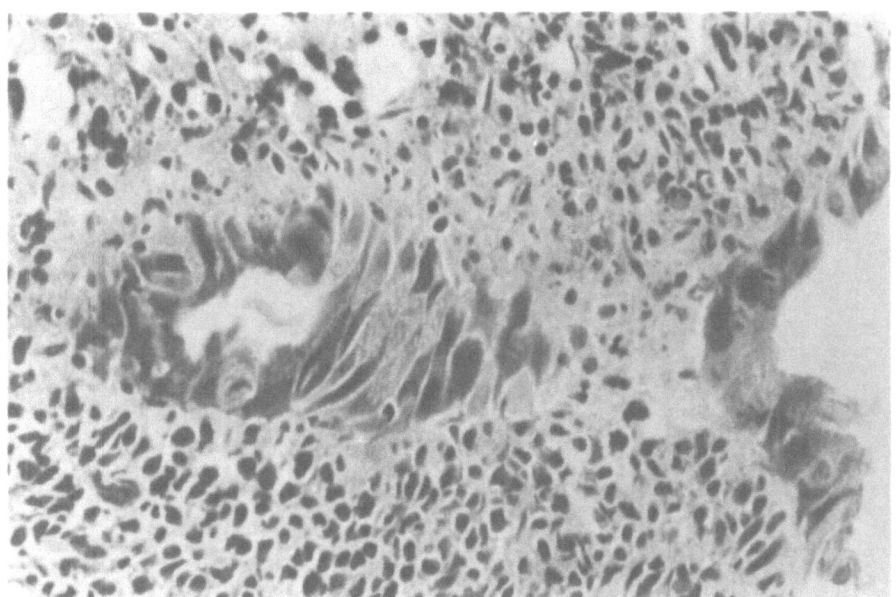

Figure 27-1 Metaplasia. Note irregularity of nuclear size.

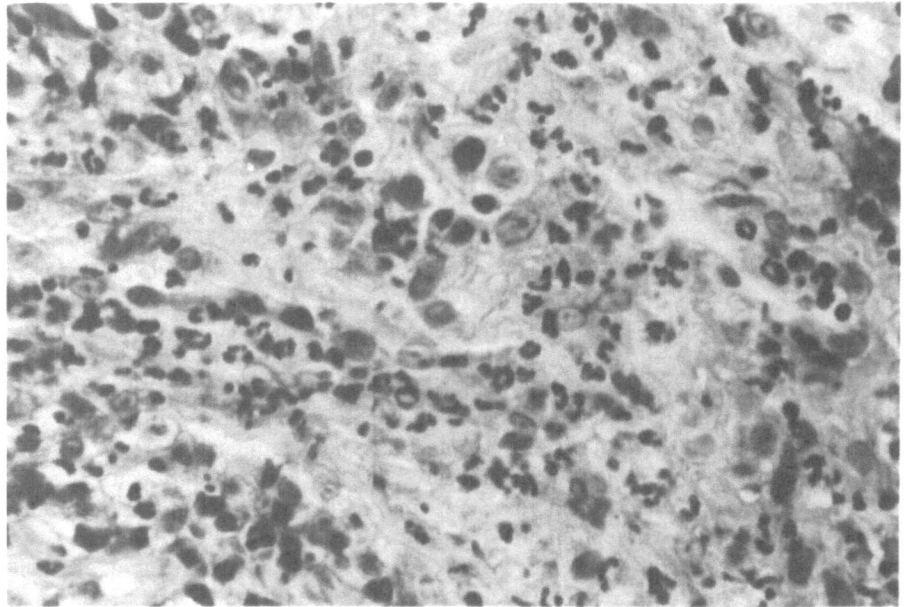

Figure 27-2   Metaplasia. Cells have irregular arrangement.

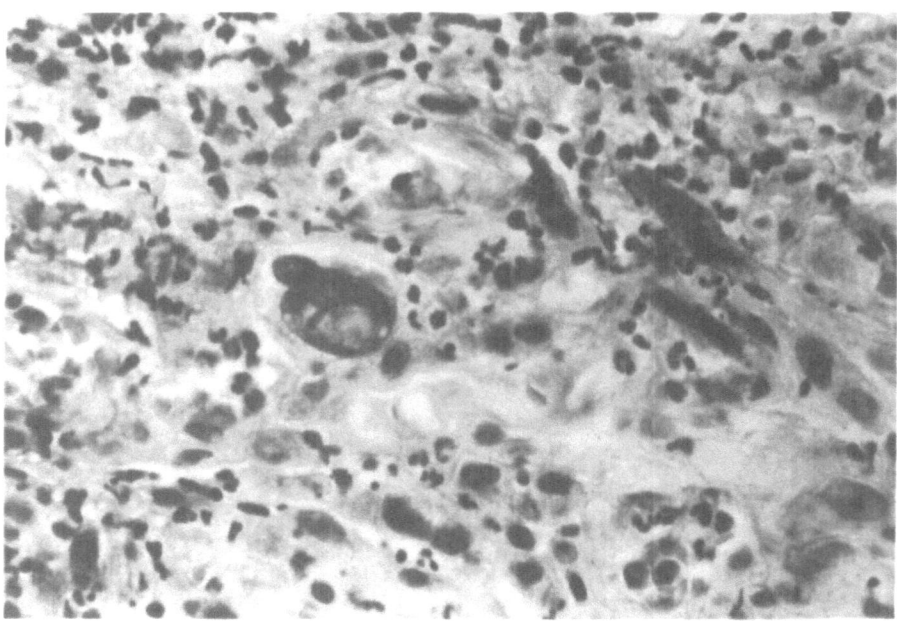

Figure 27-3   Pseudodysplasia, originally thought to be carcinoma.

Table 27-2
Some Items in the Recognition of Epithelial Dysplasia

Irregular sizes of adjacent cells
Loss of normal cell polarity
Layering or piling up of cells
Irregular sizes, shapes and chromatic contents of adjacent cells
Enlarged individual nuclei, reflecting polyploidy
Increased numbers and sizes of nucleoli
Misplaced mitoses
Sometimes cytologic acidophilia
Ultrastructural loss of cell polarity with microvilli facing stroma
Ultrastructural intracytoplasmic lacunae with microvilli
Ultrastructural irregular cell membranes and attachment sites

Table 27-3 asks some of the questions about cases of dysplasia: 1) How are inflammatory and regenerative colonic epithelial changes to be distinguished from true hyperplasia and dysplasia? This can be done by downgrading atypical changes in the presence of considerable inflammation. 2) What is the borderline between colonic hyperplasia and dysplasia? It still has to be worked out, but in the presence of inflammation, a small degree of irregularity would probably be considered regenerative hyperplasia, and not dysplasia. 3) Is all dysplasia precancerous? One can observe the distinctively different appearance of the nuclei (Figure 27-6). They are abnormally enlarged compared to the cell size. Most of them have a very prominent nucleolus, and they are irregularly piled up. This is indicative of moderate dysplasia. It occurs in an area with very little inflammation. Severe dysplasia has nowadays to be considered precancerous.

Table 27-3
Questions About Dysplasia

1. How are inflammatory and regenerative colonic epithelial changes distinguished from true hyperplasia and dysplasia?
2. What is the borderline between colonic hyperplasia and dysplasia?
3. Is all dysplasia precancerous?
4. How do we know that colonic adenomatous change is really benign neoplasia?

In another case of even more severe change, there is villous hyperplasia and some glandular proliferation within the tips of the villous fronds (Figure 27-7). At higher power, it is one of the worst looking areas (Figure 27-8). This is carcinoma in situ. Others call this in situ anaplasia. This degree of in situ anaplasia, or severe dysplasia, is genuinely precancerous.

Dr Riddell's chapter (Table 27-4) from the monograph, *Pathogenesis of Colorectal Cancer* (WB Saunders Co, 1978) tells what happened to 20 patients with moderate

Table 27-4
Outcome at the End of Follow-up in the 20 Patients in Whom One or More Biopsies Showed Moderate Dysplasia

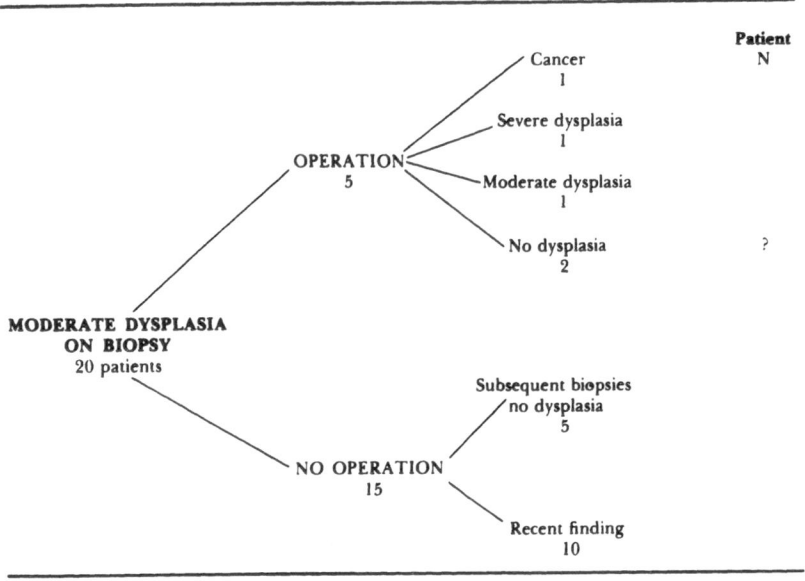

Table 27-5
Outcome at the End of Follow-up in the 13 Patients in Whom One or More Biopsies Showed Severe Dysplasia

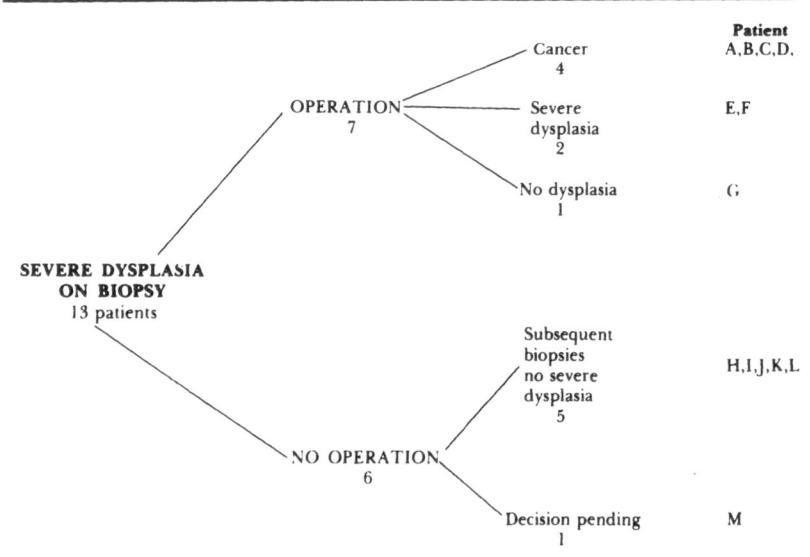

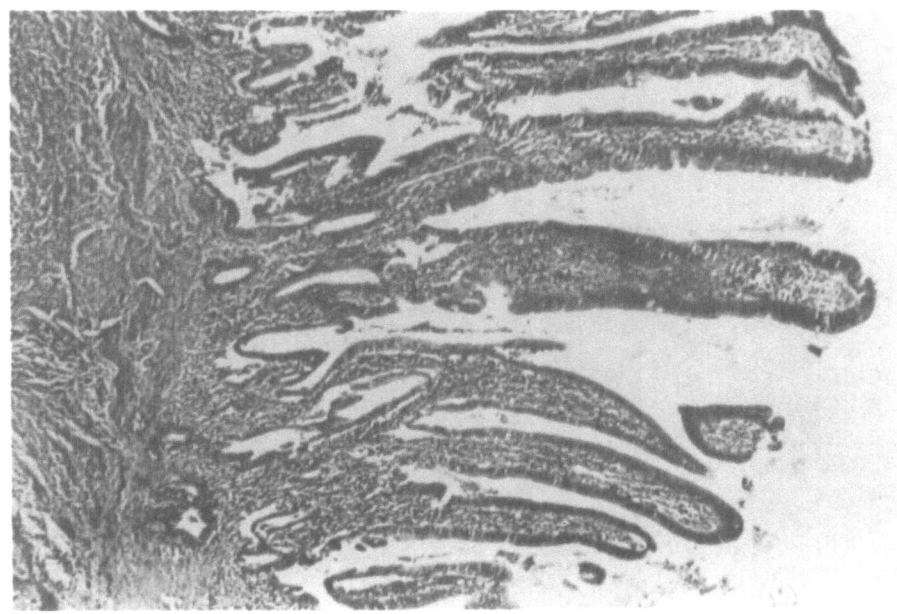

Figure 27-4 Ulcerative colitis with villous hyperplasia.

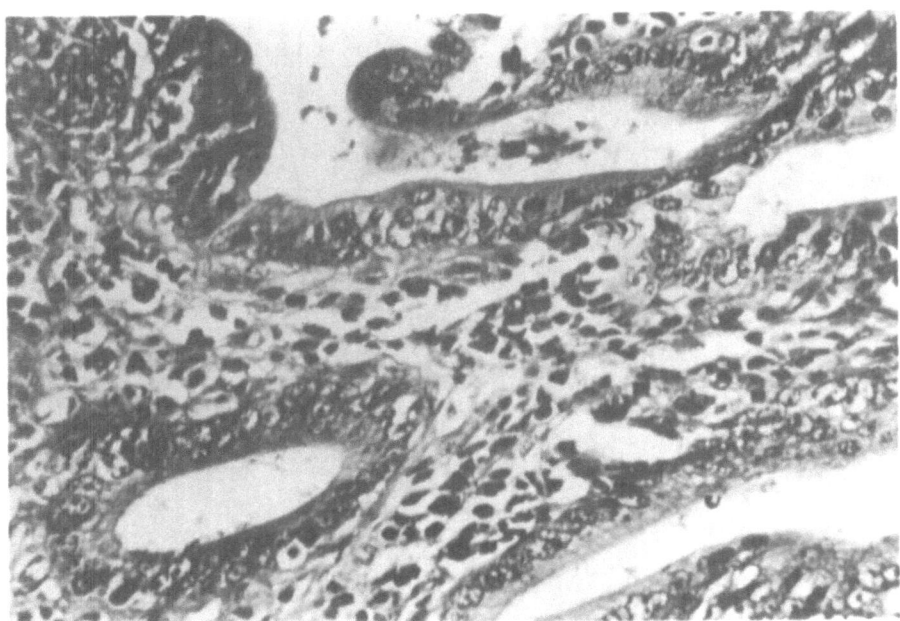

Figure 27-5 Same case as Figure 27-4. Active inflammation; insignificant atypia.

168

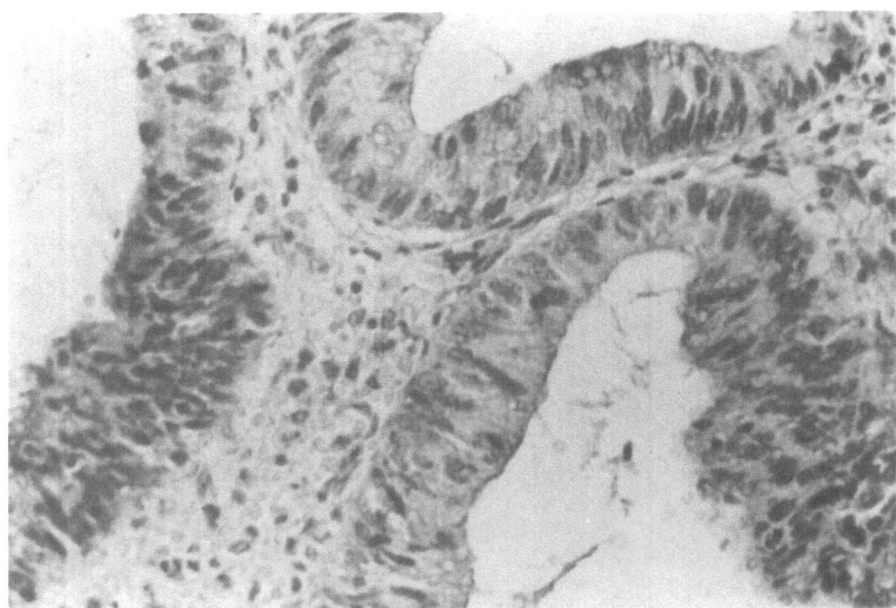

Figure 27-6 Dysplasia. Nuclei are abnormally large compared to cell size; nucleoli are prominent.

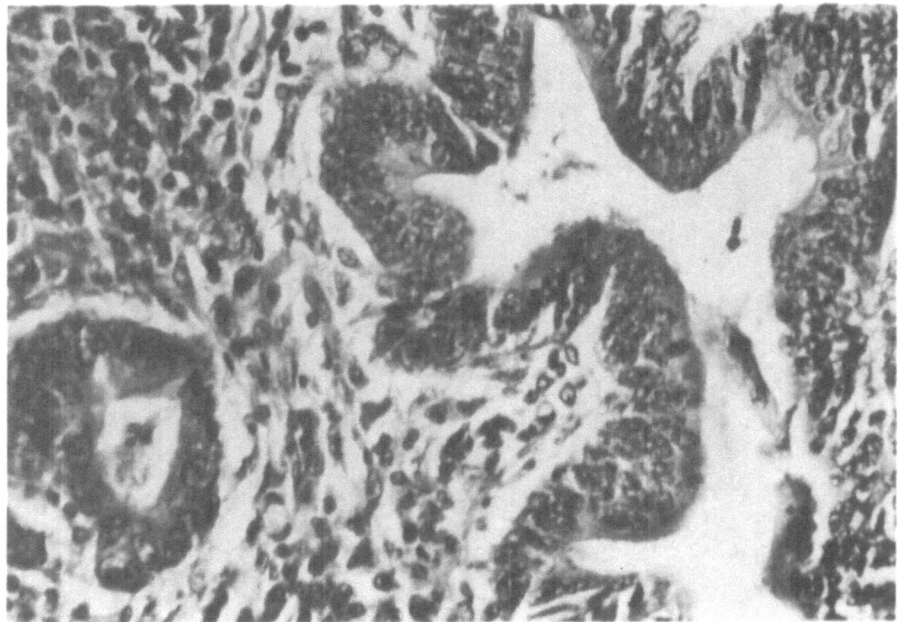

Figure 27-7 Dysplasia with villous hyperplasia and some glandular proliferation.

dysplasia. Of five patients who had an operation, one had cancer; one had severe dysplasia; one had moderate dysplasia; and two had none. At the time of colectomy, 15 of 20 patients had no operations, and five had no dysplasia subsequently. The other ten are still being studied. At the University of Chicago, the yield with moderate dysplasia on biopsy was 1 out of 20 with carcinoma.

Table 27-5 indicates what happened to 13 patients who had severe dysplasia on biopsy. Of seven who had operations, four had cancer, two still had dysplasia and one did not have any. Six of the 13 patients did not have operations. Subsequent biopsies showed no dysplasia in five, and the outcome for one patient is pending. The yield in severe dysplasia, was 4 out of 13.

Thus, out of 33 cases, there were 5 carcinomas, or about one-sixth of the patients in the two studies. One of the most important factors is the small number of cases. As yet, there is not a large enough sample upon which to base a definite conclusion in regard to the incidence of carcinoma in cases of severe dysplasia.

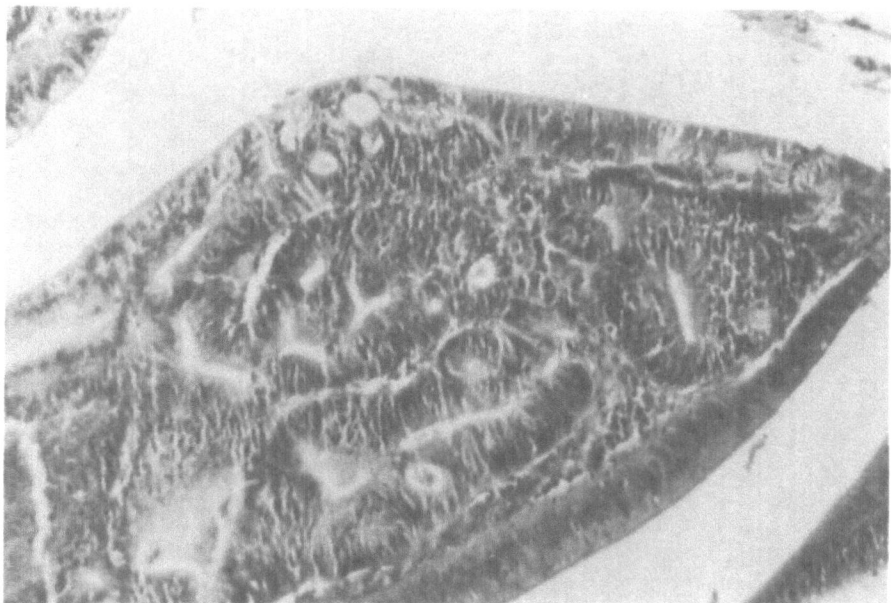

Figure 27-8 Higher power of Figure 27-7; carcinoma in situ.

Figure 27-9 shows an adenomatous polyp. It has arisen in the colon of a person with ulcerative colitis. At least 3% of the population have polyps like this. At the end of the polyp, an uninvolved base colonic epithelium may be seen. Notice how different the polyp epithelium looks from the uninvolved epithelium. At higher power (Figure 27-10), part of that polyp is seen. Adenomatous epithelium in polyps is thought to be transformed, that is, to be benign neoplastic epithelium. This is based upon tritiated thymidine uptake, the turnover rates of the cells, and ultrastructural changes. Is there any dysplasia in this adenomatous polyp? There seems to be no significant dysplasia. To answer the question, how do we know whether colonic adenomatous epithelium is

170

transformed or is neoplastic? We know it mostly by the ultrastructure and the DNA studies of tritiated thymidine uptake.

How is genuine dysplasia to be graded? You have been shown moderate and severe dysplasia, and what seems to be carcinoma in situ. It is simply degrees of change of the various cytologic atypias that have already been described. Is the extent of colonic

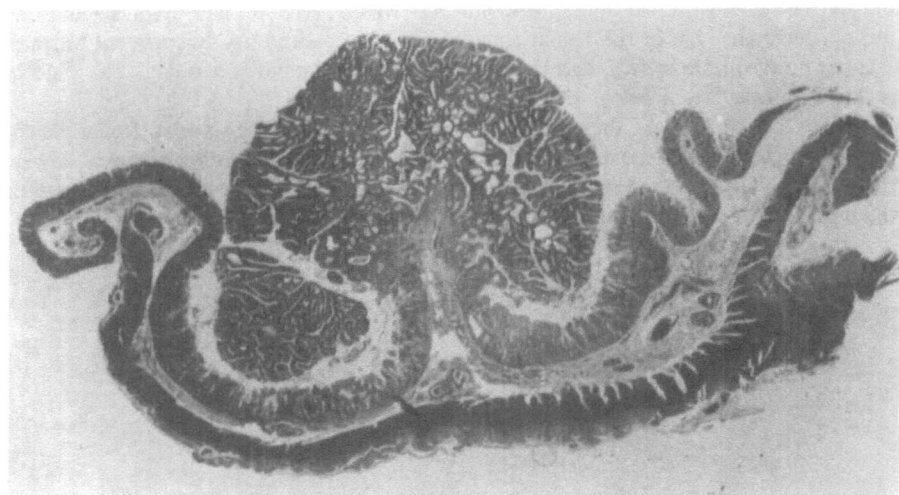

Figure 27-9   Adenomatous polyp in colon of patient with ulcerative colitis.

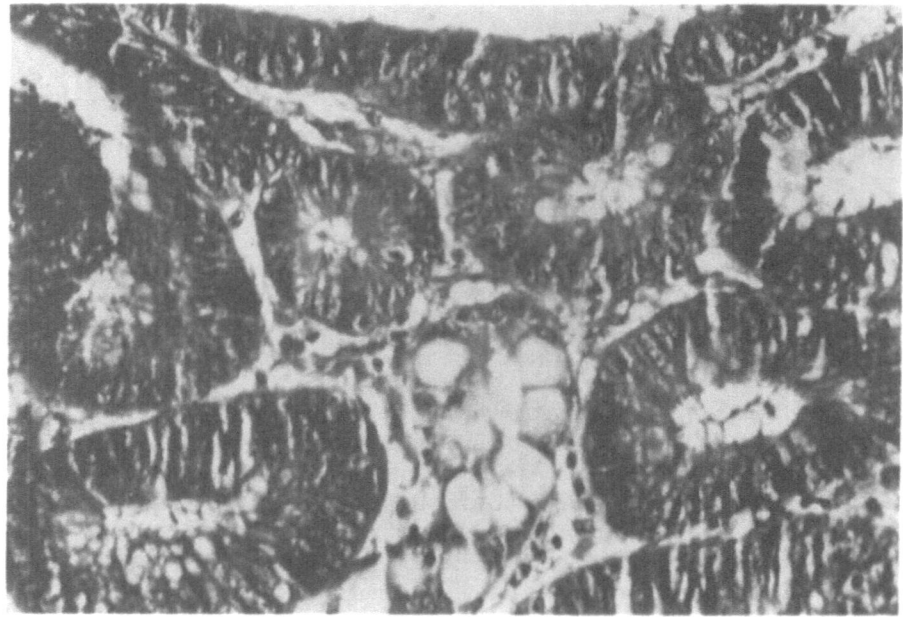

Figure 27-10   Higher power of Figure 27-9.

dysplasia more significant than its presence? This is not known, but there are some cases reported by Dr Riddell and found elsewhere in the literature, in which carcinoma of the colon and ulcerative colitis occurred when there was not any dysplasia anywhere else in the colon. In many other cases, there is dysplasia found in most areas.

How can severe dysplasia be distinguished from carcinoma in situ? Figure 27-11 shows a cancer of the colon arising from a flat surface. This would be very difficult to identify radiologically, endoscopically or in gross pathology. From time to time every laboratory has experienced a case where only the regional lymph nodes first show metastatic carcinoma. None is found in the original colon blocks, but on going back to the specimen it is found that there was, indeed, a carcinoma which was unrecognizable grossly. The carcinoma is of the unusual small cell type, and it is invading the submucosa. This border, seen under higher power, shows some glands which are not invading, and are lined by very atypical cells. Out of them come individual groups of cancer cells which invade down through the stroma (Figure 27-12). How can carcinoma in situ be identified? In the cervix and elsewhere, one of the simplest ways to identify carcinoma in situ is to find it next to an invasive carcinoma. As the criteria are sharpened by looking at the noninvasive part, it may be recognized in the absence of invasive carcinoma. How is it distinguished otherwise? It is very difficult to tell severe colonic dysplasia from carcinoma in situ, and individuals will differ in their criteria. Does genuine colonic carcinoma in situ exist? Yes, it does. It certainly exists with invasive carcinoma, and it appears to exist elsewhere as well.

How often, how rapidly, and how extensively does colonic dysplasia change into ordinary invasive carcinoma? It is not really known. It may be five or ten years from dysplasia to carcinoma, but there is no way of knowing whether the dysplasia has been found on the first day or the first month that it existed.

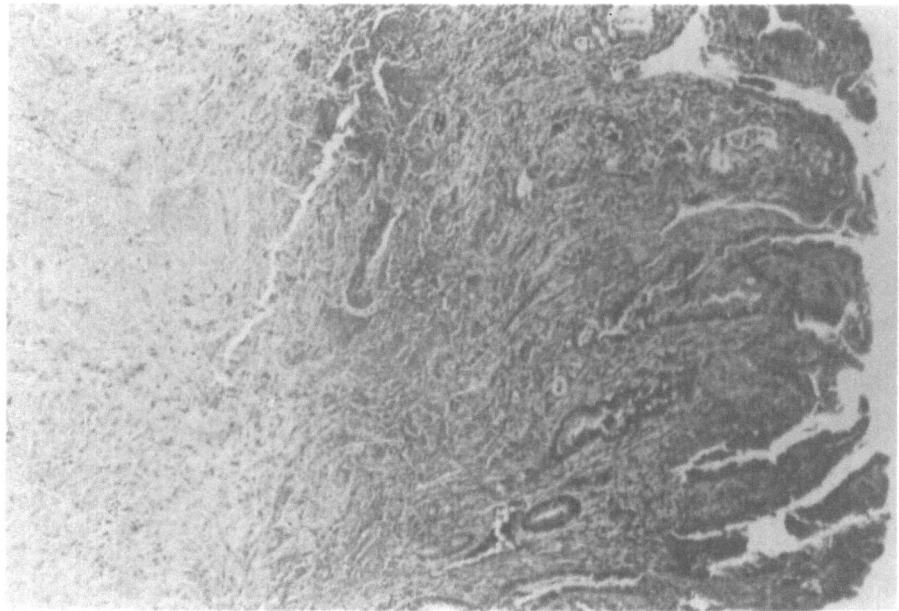

Figure 27-11 Cancer of the colon arising from a flat surface.

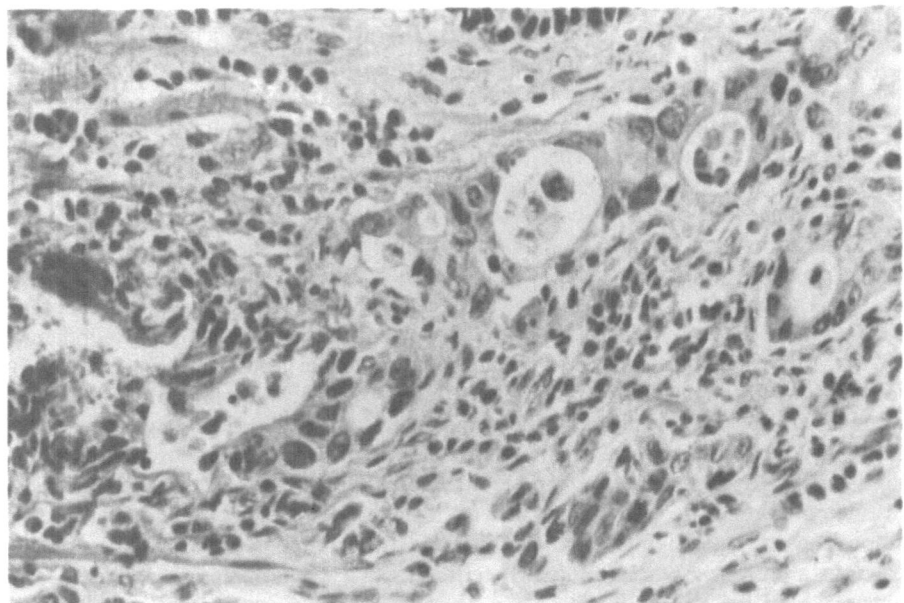

Figure 27-12 Same case as Figure 27-11. Some glands are not invasive, lined by atypical cells.

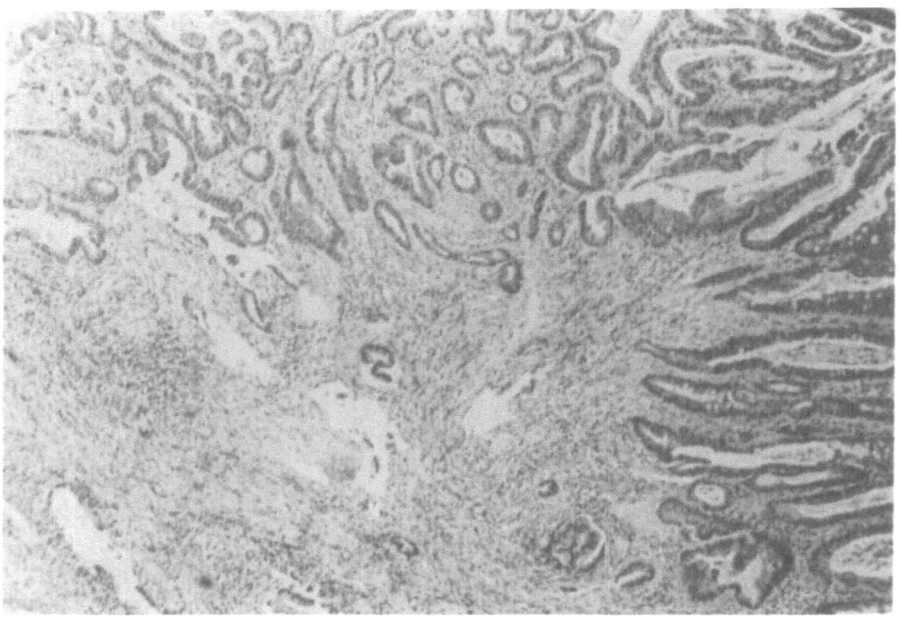

Figure 27-13 Crohn's disease; full thickness transmural inflammatory ileocolitis.

This high point is to highlight the problem of carcinoma complicating Crohn's disease. I find about 70 cases in the literature. It is not in the monograph that I referred to previously. Riddell et al consider that cancer pathogenesis does not presently involve Crohn's disease. I believe it does. Figure 27-13 shows a recent Crohn's disease case, a full thickness transmural inflammatory ileocolitis. In the cecum, there is villous hyperplasia with invasive carcinoma at the base, and elsewhere in the cecum is another little area of villous hyperplasia, just as in ulcerative colitis (Figure 27-14). In Crohn's disease, about half of the colonic carcinomas have been in the right colon, about half in the left. About 20 of the 70 cases have occurred in the ileum, either proximal to permanent ileostomies or, in quite a number of cases, in the bypassed segment. It is very difficult or impossible to diagnose by radiography or endoscopy a carcinoma arising in a bypassed segment that had regional ileitis.

Figure 27-15 shows the atypical hyperplasia or dysplasia of the villous area, and the invasive adenocarcinomatous glands extending down into the submucosa.

What does the pathologic diagnosis of colonic dysplasia mean to the clinician? Dr Farmer has been better able to tell you than I. Dr Riddel wrote that if a second biopsy again shows dysplasia, the problem should be taken seriously, and a colectomy should be considered.

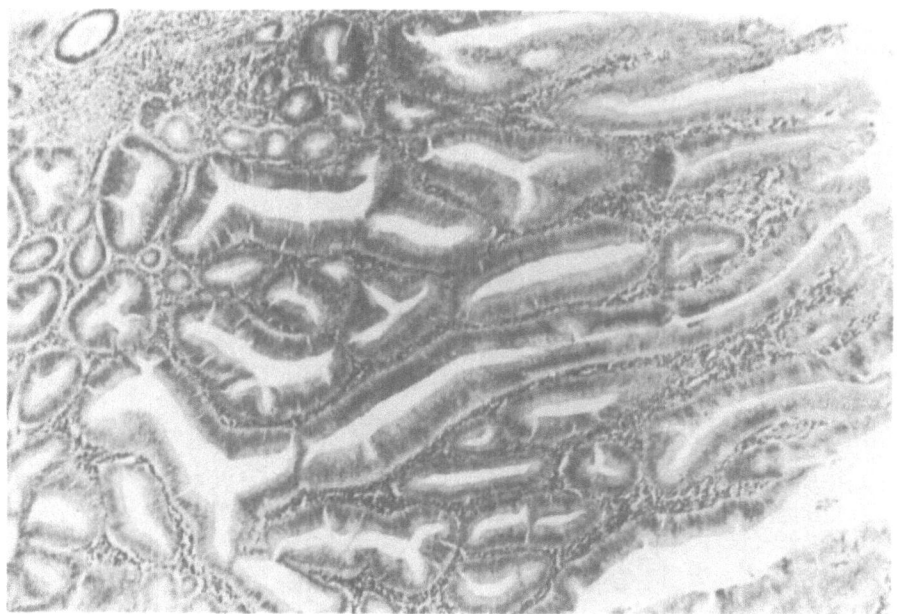

Figure 27-14   Small area of villous hyperplasia in cecum.

174

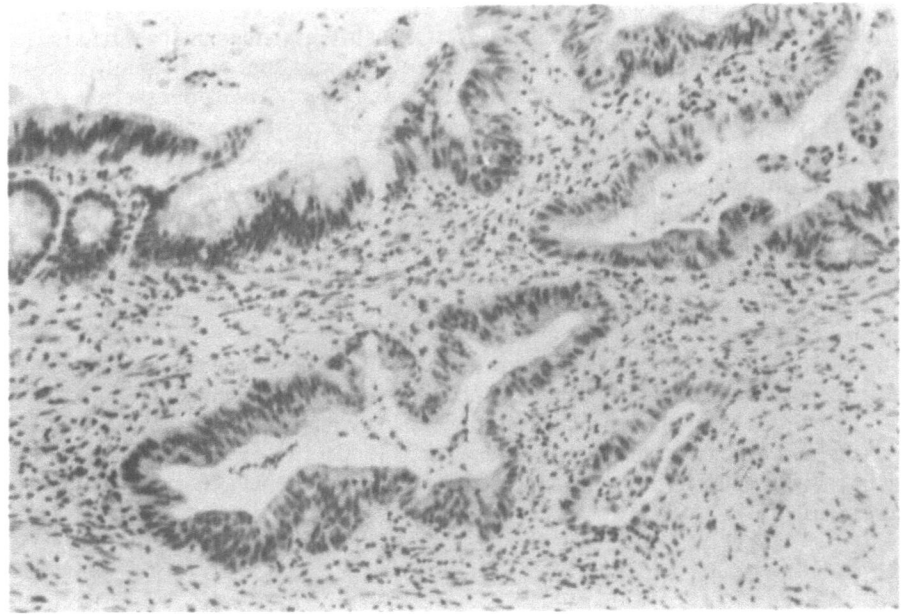

Figure 27-15 Atypical hyperplasia or dysplasia of villous area; invasive adenocarcinomatous glands extend into submucosa.

28 A Program for Management of Ulcerative Colitis with Respect to Cancer

Burton I. Korelitz, MD

In the early studies of ulcerative colitis from 1915 to 1949, we found that 60% of patients came to surgery and the mortality rate was very high, 55%. In later years the surgical rate decreased considerably so that in a relatively recent large study from 1966 to 1975, only 15% of 269 patients followed for 11 years came to surgery, with a mortality of 1%. This means that ulcerative colitis is at its very worst in the early years of the disease. If patients survive the first few years of disease, they are likely to do well.

In children, in the early years, the surgical rate was as high as 66%, with a mortality of 23%. Even though the surgical incidence has been significantly reduced in recent years, it remains at 35% with a mortality of 5%. This means that a great number of colons are resected in those early years of disease which, if left in situ, would have been vulnerable to carcinoma. Therefore, colectomies seem to have reduced the risk of cancer. However, medical therapy has improved along with the overall spectrum of the disease. The net result is more patients at risk for carcinoma, since their colons have not been removed. The only absolute indications for surgery in ulcerative colitis are perforation, sometimes exsanguinating hemorrhage, carcinoma if it is already present, and persistent dysplasia.

The relative indications for surgery are complications of the disease which are potentially reversible. Therefore, in recent years, with response to good medical therapy, many of these cases have not come to surgery. Thus they remain at risk for developing carcinoma.

The factors which have clearly been responsible for the increase in risk are: 1) the universal extent of disease, and 2) the duration, empirically starting at ten years and increasing thereafter, even though there are scattered cases occurring before ten years. We had one patient, a 16-year-old girl, who had onset at age 11. She had a subtotal colectomy at 16, and a one-foot-long carcinoma was found in the rectal segment at age 17. We are now investigating the difference between duration and age of onset as to vulnerability. Does it make any difference if the child has onset of colitis at age 7 and has the disease for 20 years, or if it starts at age 25 and lasts 20 years thereafter? The duration rather than the young age of onset may be the more important factor.

A few years ago some investigators concluded that the risk of carcinoma was so high in patients with ulcerative colitis of ten years' duration and universal disease, that they recommended prophylactic total proctocolectomy. At that time there were few diagnostic modalities for surveillance. Even left-sided ulcerative colitis is not without risk. Such patients too, are vulnerable to carcinoma but it seems to occur at a much later date than in those with universal disease.

What is the attitude of the patient for whom a total colectomy is recommended? He has already withstood the "bad" years early in the course of the disease. After ten years, he is usually in high school or college, doing well, and not likely to take kindly to a recommendation of this kind. He has learned that there is morbidity to be expected from the procedure, with possible mortality both in the immediate postoperative period and as a result of problems with the ileostomy that follow at a later date. He has to contend with a body image that includes an ileostomy. In the male there is still a small but definite risk of sexual dysfunction if he has his rectal segment removed. The physician shares the same concerns as those of his patient, but he will also be concerned whether the patient will return for surveillance which is the alternate form of protection. The physician is certainly more aware of the risk of carcinoma than is the patient.

If patients are still crippled by their ulcerative colitis after ten years of disease, they become candidates for colectomy by the usual criteria. If they are having severe recurrences of ulcerative colitis after ten years, they too are candidates for colectomy, independent of the fear of carcinoma. If these patients have strictures of the colon or rectum which cannot be adequately reached or studied by colonoscopy and biopsies, they, too, must lose their colons for reasons other than carcinoma or dysplasia. Finally, the majority is probably best represented by patients with a long history of ulcerative colitis who either refuse elective colectomy or remain unavailable for it.

These are the kinds of problems with which we can expect to deal. Dr Waye and I studied a patient with a stricture which could very well have been a carcinoma. Actually, only about one third of strictures complicating long-standing ulcerative colitis prove to be malignant, but unless the strictures can be studied adequately, they all have to be considered carcinomas until proven otherwise. This particular patient did not have a carcinoma, but unfortunately, in the course of trying to determine this, perforated during colonoscopy and lost his colon anyway. This is another risk that must be considered in the course of long-term follow-up.

Another of our cases showed a specific lesion. Despite colonoscopy and biopsies, we found no carcinoma. Nevertheless, a year later, when the examination was repeated, the stricture could not be traversed. However, tissue was biopsied and found to be consistent with dysplasia. As a result, surgery was performed and a carcinoma found.

Surveillance is advantageous because the dysplasia usually precedes the carcinoma. If we find the dysplasia, if it is a persistent finding, and if the colectomy is done, the chances are that the carcinoma can be "cured" before it develops. The likelihood of cure would be still better, if no cancer were present, but if a cancer already exists, it is more likely to be a Duke's A or B type without invasion than a more advanced lesion.

The major candidates for surveillance are those with empirically eight years of disease (rather than ten) and involvement of most of the colon. In some cases we cannot determine if the right side of the colon is involved until the colonoscopy is done and biopsies taken. The right side may never be involved, or it might be superifically involved and appear normal by x-ray and/or colonoscopy, after having been quiescent or minimally active for a long period after the early years of active disease.

The disadvantages of surveillance also have to be considered. Despite many biopsies, there could be dysplasia present without our finding it, because we are not taking biopsies from every segment of the entire colon. Dysplasia might be absent despite the existence of a carcinoma, as has been true in several of our cases. If dysplasia is absent in the rectum but present more proximally, frequent rectal biopsies without periodic colonoscopic biopsies may lead to missing it far more proximally.

Finally, we must be aware of the quality of life to which the patient is subjected when he participates in a surveillance program, even if he has no carcinoma and no dysplasia. The anxiety or chronic stress, because of fear of procedures and their outcome, represents a disease in itself for some patients.

Our current program for detection of the dysplasia and carcinoma is shown in Table 28-1. A sigmoidoscopy and rectal biopsy is performed annually after the diagnosis of ulcerative colitis has been made. If a suspicious lesion is seen, a biopsy can be taken. If no such lesions is seen, a biopsy can be taken from any region that is accessible and where bleeding can be easily controlled. This is usually done annually for the first ten years and twice a year thereafter. It is a simple procedure and complications are infrequent and of little consequence.

Table 28-1
Program for Detection of Dysplasia and Carcinoma
Complicating Ulcerative Colitis

---

1. Sigmoidoscopy and rectal biopsy
   a) annually until 10 years
   b) semi-annually after 10 years

2. Barium enema
   a) bi-annually until 10 years
   b) bi-annually after 10 years (alternating with colonoscopy)*

3. Colonoscopy and multiple biopsies
   a) bi-annually after 10 years (alternating with barium enema)*

4. Colonic washing for cytology after 10 years (when available)

5. Serial CEA levels (experimental)

---

*More frequently if disease is active.

As far as the barium enema is concerned, this should be done annually up until ten years if there is ulcerative colitis activity. One must weigh the risk of over-radiation against the possibility of the carcinoma complicating ulcerative colitis. The latter risk is much higher than the theoretical risk of provoking a carcinoma from radiation.

If, in the first ten years, the disease is quiescent, a barium enema should not be done as often, but certainly if there is low-grade activity. Beginning at the ten-year mark, or even the eight-year mark in some, colonoscopy with multiple biopsies should be done. Whether this should be done annually or every other year will be influenced to some extent by the clinical severity and whether there is a specific lesion such as early stricture formation. In the "average" case, colonoscopy with multiple biopsies and the barium enema can be alternated. However, if the index of suspicion increases, both the barium enema and the colonoscopy with multiple biopsies should be performed annually.

There are other diagnostic techniques for surveillance. Colonic washings for cytology may be very helpful. Theoretically, CEA levels should be a boon to this particular problem, particularly if a baseline is obtained early in the course of the ulcerative colitis, with annual CEA levels thereafter.

To solve the problems of surveillance, we need as many retrospective and prospective studies as possible of the patients at highest risk and of those clinical situations in which the dysplasia has already been found in order to plan meaningful programs.

BIBLIOGRAPHY

Banks BM, Korelitz BI, Zetzel L: The course of non-specific ulcerative colitis: review of twenty years' experience and late results. *Gastroenterology* 32:983–1012, 1957.

deDombal FT, Watts JM, Watkinson G, et al: Local complications of ulcerative colitis: stricture, pseudopolyposis and carcinoma of the colon and rectum. *Br Med J* 1:1442–1447, 1966.

DeVroede GJ, Taylor WF, Sauer WG, et al: Cancer risk and life expectancy of children with ulcerative colitis. *N Engl J Med* 285:17–21, 1971.

DeVroede G, Taylor WF: On calculating cancer risk and survival of ulcerative colitis patients and the life table method. *Gastroenterology* 71:505–509, 1976.

Dobbins WO: Current status of the precancer lesion in ulcerative colitis. *Gastroenterology* 73:1431–1433, 1977.

Edwards FS, Truelove SC: Course and prognosis of ulcerative colitis. IV. Carcinoma of the colon. *Gut* 5:15–22, 1964.

Korelitz BI, Gribetz D, Danziger I: The prognosis of ulcerative colitis with onset in childhood. 1. The pre-steroid era. *Ann Intern Med* 57:582–591, 1962.

Lennard-Jones JE, Morson BC, Ritchie JK, et al: Cancer in colitis: assessment of the individual risk by clinical and histological criteria. *Gastroenterology* 73:1280–1289, 1977.

Levin B, Riddel RH, Kirsner JB: Management of precancerous lesions of the gastrointestinal tract. *Clin Gastroenterol* 5:827–853, 1976.

MacDougall IPM: The cancer risk in ulcerative colitis. *Lancet* 2:655–658, 1964.

Michener WM, Gage RP, Sauer WG, et al: The prognosis of chronic ulcerative colitis in childhood. *N Engl J Med* 265:1075–1079, 1961.

Morson BC, Pang LSC: Rectal biopsy as an aid to cancer control in ulcerative colitis. *Gut* 8:423–434, 1967.

Proceedings of the Pathology Conference, National Foundation for Ileitis and Colitis, Inc, Tarrytown, NY, October 29–30, 1977, *Session II: Neoplasia and Inflammatory Bowel Disease.*

PANEL DISCUSSION

Question: 1. Is there any role for the flexible sigmoidoscope in surveillance? 2. Do you recommend proplylactic total colectomy after ten years of universal ulcerative colitis?

Dr Korelitz: My endoscopy colleagues have taught me that if it is worth doing colonoscopy at all, why stop at the splenic flexure? Cover the entire colon! Certainly the dysplasia can occur anywhere within the colon. Therefore, I prefer passing the colonoscope to the cecum if possible.

As far as removing everyone's colon after ten years, we believe most patients will not accept this. They do not want to sacrifice their colons. Usually, by that time they are no longer symptomatic, and it is difficult for the intelligent patient to reconcile a recommendation for total colectomy even though it is presented to them in a rational and logical manner. The patients themselves have solved that problem for us and it makes the program of surveillance all the more essential.

Dr Farmer: The value of performing a total colonoscopy as opposed to fiberoptic sigmoidoscopy is twofold. In the first place, there is at least the theoretical consideration that if the mucosa is biopsied in various locations in the colon with multiple sequential biopsies, the chances of finding dysplasia are greater than if one simply does rectal or distal colon biopsies. This still has to be proved statistically. When we are considering a high risk population, a total colonoscopy should be done. I think fiberoptic sigmoidoscopy is a valuable technical procedure, but not for cancer surveillance for ulcerative colitis. If we develop a logical system for surveillance, if a definition of dysplasia can be universally accepted, and if there is statistical significance established, then the risk factors can be defined. This has been an important contribution of colonoscopy.

Question: I would like Dr Waye to comment on the case of stricture complicating ulcerative colitis that perforated during colonoscopy, particularly in the light of the frequency of malpractice suits?

Dr Waye: This was one of the first colonoscopies that I had done in a patient with inflammatory bowel disease. The long stricture in the sigmoid colon was one of two strictures, and I was quite eager to look at both. That was before we had small instruments able to go through strictures. I was much more eager a colonoscopist, than I now am. Now when I come upon a stricture that does not appear to be passable with a regular sized endoscope, I do not attempt to get through it. This is the only complication I have had in performing several hundred colonoscopies on patients with inflammatory bowel disease. The complication rate is rather low. In fact, when talking to endoscopists who perform many colonoscopies in patients with inflammatory bowel disease, the risk of complication is relatively low. It is low because we now realize nothing can be gained by attempting to force one's way through a stricture or reaching inaccessible areas.

Yes, there are lawsuits in progress in New York, and all of us are aware of colleagues who have been involved in malpractice suits.

Question: In a patient with inflammatory bowel disease how do you determine whether it is only proctosigmoiditis and not more proximal disease? If a patient is seen with what appears to be proctosigmoiditis with a negative barium enema, how does the panel feel about colonoscopy at the time of the original diagnosis with regard to consideration of future effect?

Dr Waye: Our definition of proctosigmoiditis is a relatively negative one, namely a normal barium enema; in other words, a radiographic definition with an abnormal sigmoidoscopic examination. With the advent of colonoscopy, we are now able to get above the inflamed mucosa and this is one area in which we are using fiberoptic sigmoidoscopy. We never made a positive diagnosis of proctosigmoiditis without following the patient to make sure that more extensive disease was not missed. There were certainly cases in which we believed the diagnosis was proctosigmoiditis when, in fact, it was total colon disease, but the changes were subtle or early and were not picked up by conventional means. This is another area in which endoscopy can be valuable. I do not feel that total colonoscopy is necessary in all cases of proctosigmoiditis, but I think this is a good illustration of where fiberoptic sigmoidoscopy for a distance of 50, 60, or 70 cm is valuable to be certain that there is normal mucosa above the level of inflamed mucosa. This finding correlates statistically with a good prognosis.

Question: Do you prepare ulcerative colitis patients for endoscopy in the same way you prepare a nonulcerative colitis patient?

Dr Waye: No. We are very reluctant to use laxatives, and the preparation has to be tailored to the patient. Very briefly, if the patient is having more than four loose bowel movements per day, we give them no cathartics but only a liquid diet for 48 hours and enemas. If they are in a phase where they are recovering from an acute disease, even if they are having one or two bowel movements per day, we do not prescribe cathartics for fear of exacerbating the disease. If they are having less than four stools per day, we recommend 5 to 10 ounces of citrate of magnesia and enemas.

Question: If you get a report of dysplasia, particularly if it is moderate to severe, what course of action do you take? Are you saying that any patient with ulcerative colitis, regardless of age of onset and extent, should go into a program of surveillance after 8 to 10 years, or are there exceptions?

Dr Korelitz: The answer to the first question is relatively easy because all instances to date of dysplasia found on surveillance have been found on rectal biopsies. Therefore, if we find it, we repeat the rectal biopsy to see if it is still there. The only time we found dysplasia on colonoscopic biopsies was when the procedure was done for that specific lesion in a stricture. Dysplasia has not yet been discovered in random surveys. This contrasts with the experience of other institutions.

The answer to the second question is *yes.* After 8 to 10 years of universal (or what appears to be close to universal) disease, the program must start. Whether you tell the patient that it is a program, or whether you just do it, depends on the physician-patient relationship.

Dr Gelernt: I agree with Dr Farmer. Who accepts surgery and who does not is very much dependent on the physician's attitude to surgery.

I have a question about surveillance: Who should be the final evaluator of the data that is obtained at surveillance? In the past year we have seen over a dozen patients with carcinoma, many already having significant metastatic disease at the time of surgery. I am troubled by some of the things that were shown this morning. One is a slide of a patient with serial barium enema x-rays, one year apart. The second one shows an obvious contour defect, and yet the patient went on to have colonoscopy. Had this patient not had ulcerative colitis and had a barium enema, with that significant a contour defect there would be no question of the diagnosis. I think that the people doing the surveillance after ten years of following the same patient are so emotionally involved that they have a great deal of difficulty recommending surgery to a patient whom they feel they have "saved" from surgery for 10 years. I think perhaps it might be a good idea if a gastroenterologist, after obtaining data at the end of ten years, would "trade" the patient with a colleague. The colleague could act as a consultant and suggest a decision. We would have far fewer patients coming to surgery with metastatic disease.

Question: Dr Waye, I wonder if you could expand a bit more on what level of activity of colitis would make you refrain from doing a colonoscopy.

Dr Waye: Very briefly, most of the patients with long-standing ulcerative colitis who have their colons after ten years are not very active. Those patients who have had severe active disease for ten years have usually already lost their colons, so we are really not that concerned with the very active patient going on to long-term surveillance. I think it is difficult to obtain meaningful biopsies from patients with active inflammatory disease universally distributed, so we do have a problem. I do not like to submit patients to colonoscopy who are very active. Along that same line, I shall ask Dr Sommers a question, since he said that pathologists downgraded the significance of dysplasia when found in inflamed bowel. Do patients with inflammation of the bowel not get carcinoma just as often? How can you downplay the significance of dysplasia in certain patients who are active and then pay more significance to it than in others?

Question: What has active inflammation got to do with increase in dsyplasia?

Dr Sommers: In microscopic fields with active inflammation, the epithelial changes are not very convincing. In adjacent areas where there is less or no inflammation, the same epithelial changes would be regarded as serious.

Question: How long should one continue sulfasalazine therapy in a patient who has been treated for active colitis and is in a quiescent phase?

Dr Farmer: This is a difficult question, because it is difficult to obtain good data due to the problems of long-term studies and variations in patients. It is not a good idea to keep patients on medications forever, so I would tend to stop the medication after clinical signs of complete remission have been maintained for approximately two years. I might want to perform colonoscopy during that time. It would depend on the age of the patient, severity, previous complications, and other factors.

Dr Korelitz: I believe that once sulfasalazine has been shown to be successful in any one patient with ulcerative colitis, it should never be stopped. The complications of this drug occur early. If they do not occur in the first few months, they probably will never occur. Therefore, if the patient is maintained free of disease with sulfasalazine, the drug should be continued indefinitely.

Question: Should steroids be continued for long terms? Both Dr Farmer and Dr Korelitz suggested only short-term steroids for patients with ulcerative colitis? I am also concerned about dysplasia, not the positive diagnosis of dysplasia, but the absence of dysplasia.

Dr Sommers: Consultation is available everywhere. I use consultation for all cases of colonic dysplasia.

Dr Farmer: I think that in the patient with ulcerative colitis, on chronic steroids, the mere mentioning of reduction of steroids causes the symptoms to get worse (malnutrition, diarrhea, and rectal bleeding). This is, of course, dependent on the circumstances and the duration of treatment. Thus, if the patient is dependent on steroids, I think colectomy should be seriously considered.

Dr Korelitz: In some cases I would consider using mercaptopurine even in ulcerative colitis. We have not had double-blind studies in ulcerative colitis but, from personal experience, many patients, particularly children, have done extremely well.

Dr Farmer: I no longer agree with such a course of action. Fifteen years ago we were involved in a study of this type of case. We found that only approximately half of the patients did reasonably well. In that group of 29 patients, almost all subsequently required surgery. Because of the cancer problem, the improvements in surgical technique, the ability of patients to tolerate an ileostomy, the Kock pouch, and a variety of other factors, colectomy may be preferable to immunosuppressives in ulcerative colitis.

Dr Schmerin: I would tend to agree with Dr Korelitz. In following some of his patients, I have seen a good clinical response in patients who have been given mercaptopurine with minimal side effects and significant improvement.

Dr Waye: In general not many physicians are using mercaptopurine for ulcerative colitis. Dr Korelitz is using it in some patients but as yet we do not have any definite answers.

Question: Dr Bayless mentioned that he continues steroid treatment in children with Crohn's disease and sometimes keeps them on alternate-day steroids for 2 to 3 years. Is this because he is treating Crohn's disease, or is it because he is using alternate-day therapy? Can you use alternate-day therapy in ulcerative colitis for long periods?

Dr Korelitz: If we use minimal doses and alternate-day therapy, and the children are really doing very well, then I would not consider introducing mercaptopurine.

Dr Waye: Dr Schmerin, to get back to a question that everybody is concerned about, although toxic dilatation is not a very common problem in patients with ulcerative colitis, you mentioned that Binder said that 30% of the patients were treated medically, 40% were operated on, and 30% died. What percentage of patients at Lenox Hill Hospital are actually operated on, what percentage die, and what percentage are treated medically?

Dr Schmerin: Initially, all patients are treated medically. In reviewing our experience with 12 cases, none of the patients died and four were operated on after intensive medical therapy. Two had toxic dilatation for more than a week, and one still has toxic dilatation but is doing very well and is asymptomatic.

Dr Waye: Our incidence of emergency surgery here is low. We rarely perform total proctocolectomy for the acute phase of toxic dilatation.

Question: Can toxic megacolon persist longer than a week and still respond to a program of medical management?

Dr Korelitz: Yes, occasionally. I remember seeing a patient where the condition started as a toxic megacolon and the toxicity was relieved, but the flat film of the abdomen showed persistence of the megacolon. The patient was discharged in good condition after two months.

Question: Do you think this is more likely to occur in the patient who has Crohn's disease rather than ulcerative colitis?
Dr Korelitz: Yes.

Question: How do you survey a patient with only limited or left-sided disease?
Dr Korelitz: They are surveyed with less intensity than those with universal disease. If the patient was asymptomatic, a maximal program would be a colonoscopy and a barium enema in alternate years.
Dr Waye: There are some data to indicate that patients with limited disease have a lesser incidence of carcinoma than those with total disease, but the lesser incidence of carcinoma is proportional to the amount of colon that is involved. Those patients with left-sided disease do not have the same incidence of carcinoma as the general population. Their incidence of carcinoma is increased, but is not as high as those with universal disease.

Question: Is there any evidence that the risk of carcinoma increases with repeated barium enemas?
Dr Waye: No, it is just a feeling that we have. I would like to ask Dr Farmer his idea of what surveillance should be. Does it include a barium enema every year or every other year?
Dr Farmer: In long-standing ulcerative colitis, the barium enema appearance often becomes rather fixed. There is a loss of haustral markings and a rather tube-like colon. If one takes x-rays every year, one sees relatively few changes. Therefore, I believe that colonoscopy is far more advantageous and, in fact, becomes a "competitive" rather than a complementary procedure with barium enema under these circumstances. With colonoscopy one can see lesions but can also do the mucosal biopsies as well.
Dr Korelitz: The x-ray taken two years later can show one area that is a little bit narrower than it was. I can show it to you and say "there is where I want extra biopsies." That has paid off in our experience.

Question: In regard to toxic dilatation in pregnancy, is there ever an indication for elective termination of the pregnancy if toxic dilatation occurs early?
Dr Schmerin: I think it depends on the outcome of the dilatation. I would manage the toxic dilatation just as if the patient were not pregnant. If the patient responds medically, I would not abort the pregnancy. If the patient needs surgery because of the toxic megacolon, the risk concerns the patient herself and not the pregnancy.

Question: You do not feel that termination of the pregnancy is part of the treatment?
Dr Schmerin: That is a very difficult problem. I do not think there is enough experience with this complication to conclude that therapeutic abortion at that point would

serve to reverse the disease process. Pregnancy per se will not affect the outcome of the toxic dilatation, but I suspect the toxic dilatation and the severity of the illness of the patient will probably affect the outcome of the pregnancy. The patient will probably abort spontaneously if the disease process does not respond to medical management.

29 Why is There a Foundation for Patients with Inflammatory Bowel Disease?

Irving A. Rubin

Why is there a foundation for patients with inflammatory bowel disease (IBD)? One of the most important reasons is to focus the attention of the medical profession on the seriousness of these diseases and the problems they present to the patient.

For years there was a curtain of silence surrounding ileitis and colitis. Until 12 years ago, knowledge of IBD was stagnant; research was almost nonexistent; seminars such as today's were almost nonexistent; and papers at medical meetings were few and far between. Those working in the field had a feeling they were in a vacuum. In fact, those physicians and scientists interested in the problems of IBD could probably be counted on the fingers of two hands.

And yet, 12 short years later, because of a foundation for patients with IBD — because of the National Foundation for Ileitis and Colitis — there is much greater research activity to improve treatment and determine the cause and cure of ileitis and colitis. As a result of NFIC funding, greater research activity has been stimulated. The federal government has taken a more aggressive role in this area, more private foundations are interested in IBD, and universities are encouraging more research in this area.

Today there is more communication than ever among those in the field. The NFIC has served as a catalyst in bringing together researchers, gastroenterologists, basic scientists, and clinicians.

Improper or delayed diagnosis by primary care physicians once caused needless suffering for many patients with ileitis and colitis. Early diagnosis is becoming more the rule than the exception.

While still far from ideal, the transfer of knowledge from the laboratory to the clinic has been accelerated as the direct result of the NFIC. It is known that a certain critical mass is needed before significant results occur. Our worth has been and continues to be in stimulating the development of that critical mass.

Patients with ileitis and colitis pose a serious challenge to the physician, for they frequently need the kind of therapeutic support that goes beyond clinical treatment. Another reason for an NFIC is to provide that support – to provide the feeling that the patient is not alone, to help him understand the why and how of his disease, and to provide some answers for the patient and his family.

For many years the American public was ignorant about ileitis and colitis. Upon diagnosis, patients were devastated with fear and anxiety. I recall the confusion and uncertainty my wife and I felt when we were told our daughter had ileitis. That was 16 years ago. Today, NFIC pamphlets, written by distinguished gastroenterologists, explain the diseases in easy langulage and answer the hundreds of questions most frequently asked by patients.

The pain, embarrassment, and feelings of isolation caused by the symptoms of ileitis and colitis have damaged the family relationships and ruined the careers of many patients. Now patients can meet with those who understand their problems at NFIC Chapter meetings, and direct questions to the expert physicians who speak at such educational seminars.

The value of establishing the feeling that the patient and his family are in an empathetic and sympathetic environment cannot be underestimated. The hope provided by meeting and speaking with those who have experienced or are experiencing your problem can be a powerful stimulus for patient improvement. A physician once said to me that he thought of the NFIC as another treatment modality – an opportunity to provide help for his patient and family which went beyond his knowledge of medicine and drugs.

It is estimated there are approximately two million patients with IBD in the United States. These patients need:

1. An ombudsman or consumer advocate.
2. An organization to encourage continued research.
3. An organization to stimulate involvement by the federal government (financial funding).
4. An organization to sponsor professional education.
5. An environment in which patients can function with minimal embarrassment and prejudice in terms of schooling and career opportunities.

To this end our foundation is filling the need. Allow me to comment on our accomplishments in making the government and general public more aware of IBD. The NFIC has always played an active role in educating the government. We were part of the effort to have the National Institute of Arthritis, Metabolism and Digestive Diseases established; as well as the National Commission on Digestive Diseases, and we are now actively working with many physicians to implement the report of the National Commission on Digestive Diseases.

Twelve years ago, who would have believed that ileitis and colitis would be discussed on television and radio? Through our Chapters we have sponsored television discussions on IBD. Our commercials are being aired regularly.

Our progress so far has been made possible by hundreds of people, lay and professional. We think of ourselves as a partnership between the laity and physicians.

30 What Problems Lie Ahead for a Patient With an Ileostomy?

Margaret M. Roche, RN, ET

The Bill of Rights, published by the United Ostomy Association, is very relevant. It states that the ostomate shall:

1. Be given preoperative counseling
2. Have an appropriately positioned stoma
3. Have a well-constructed stoma
4. Have skilled postoperative nursing care
5. Have emotional support
6. Have individual instruction
7. Be informed as to the availability of supplies
8. Be provided with information on community resources
9. Have posthospital follow-up and life-long supervision
10. Benefit from team efforts of the health care professionals.

As soon as the physician realizes that the patient is to have an ileostomy, he should discuss with the patient and with the spouse or other family member, details of what is going to happen and the significance of having an ileostomy. The patient must be told what a stoma is, that it will protrude from the abdominal wall, and that this is where feces will exit from the body after the rectum has been removed. It must be recognized that the construction of a stoma can cause a drastically altered body image. The individual is not being hospitalized for a brief operative experience such as an appendectomy, after which he will go home and talk about it casually. A patient in this situation is one who may be frustrated and even devastated by his disease process and proposed surgery.

The handling of these factors by the health care team can make a significant difference between a smooth adjustment or an extremely difficult one. Most of the patients subjected to ileostomy have suffered for many years with ulcerative colitis or Crohn's disease. By the time they come to surgery they have become weakened and debilitated, and their lives have been seriously affected by the disease process. They have had multiple hospitalizations. They may be drained physically and emotionally, and have failed to respond to conventional modalities of treatment.

Employment opportunities may have been lost because of their inflammatory bowel disease (IBD). Socioeconomically they may have been rendered poverty stricken. Many patients have become so dependent on bathrooms that they know their locations wherever they are traveling. Family life may have been disrupted. In the face of such emotional trauma they are now confronted with an adjustment to an altered body image.

The enterostomal therapist has an important function to provide as a member of the health care team. The patient should be informed that an enterostomal therapist is available who will insure total rehabilitation. The patient should be seen by the enterostomal therapist prior to operation. The therapist should be briefed by the surgeon prior to the initial visit. The patient's state of knowledge of the disease and the proposed surgery should be made known to the therapist. This preoperative visit is necessary in order to build up a rapport and a relationship between the therapist and the patient. This gives the therapist a chance to evaluate the patient and establish a program of instruction and reassurance, which begins prior to the operation and continues through the postoperative period and following discharge from the hospital. Details about the patient's background, his knowledge of the disease, his feelings about the disease, and his feelings about the surgery are important.

The enterostomal therapist can contribute much to these patients, helping them understand their disease and adjust to their new state following surgery, thus allowing them to enjoy a comfortable life following the construction of an ileostomy.

It is important for the therapist in conjunction with the surgeon to select a suitable site for the stoma. Figure 30-1 depicts a well constructed stoma. It protrudes approximately one-half inch. There are at least four inches of peristomal skin in good condition surrounding the stoma. Patients with stomas such as this are easy to care for. Problems with appliances are rare. These patients may need only an annual examination. The follow-up visits may result in certain modifications due to changes in weight. Skin problems are uncommon. The stoma is healthy, red, moist and glistening.

In selecting a stoma site it is important to avoid scars, skin creases, the umbilicus, and boney prominences. These may interfere with subsequent appliance care. The stoma should be brought through the rectus abdominus muscle. The site must be selected with the patient lying, sitting, and standing.

The operative procedure with proper placement, adequate abdominal wall aperture for the ileum, avoidance of tension, fixation of the mesentery, and the use of an everted

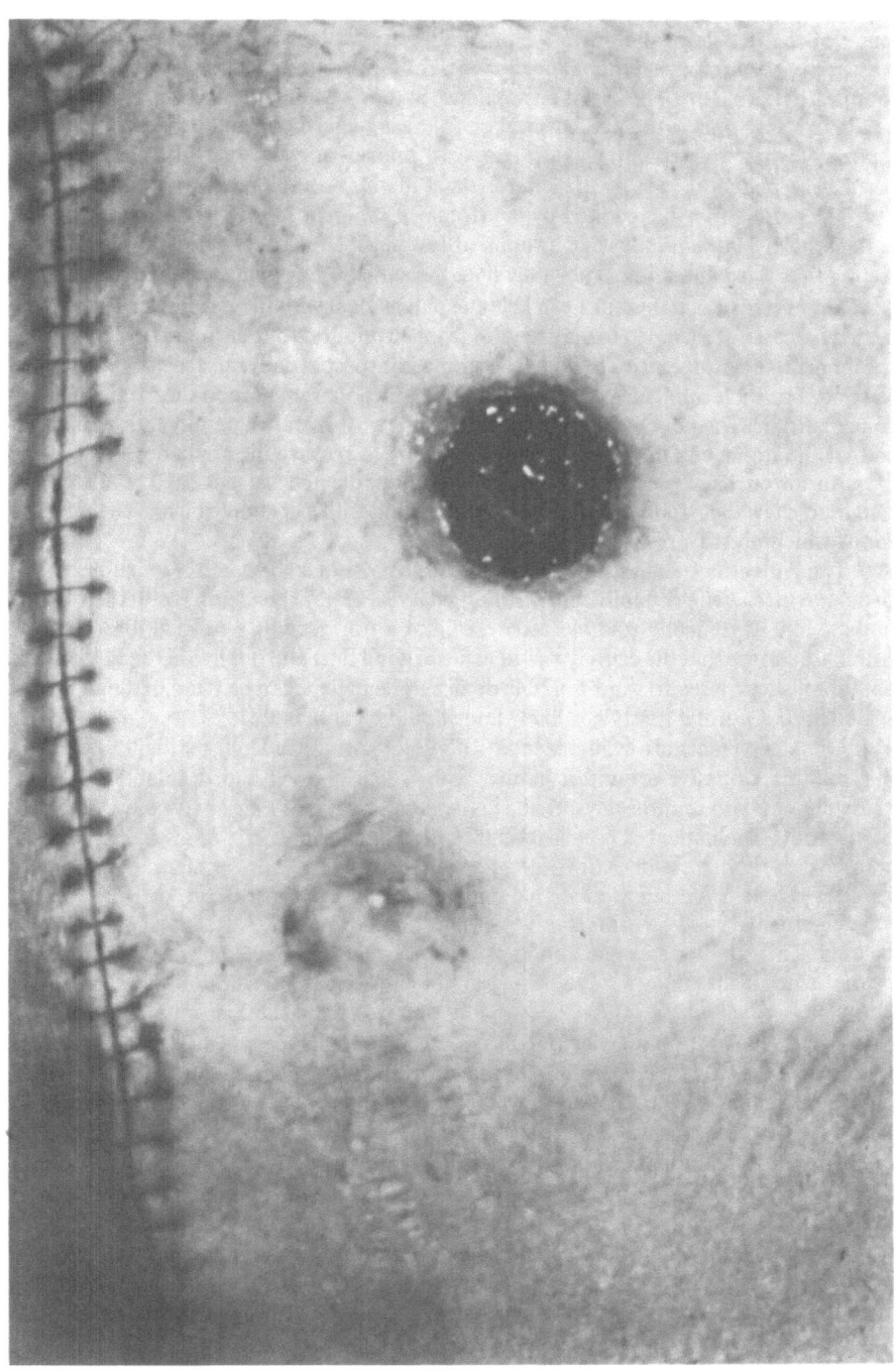

Figure 30-1 Well-constructed stoma.

stoma with primary suture of intestinal wall to skin, are all important. Preoperatively, many of the details of the operative procedure are explained to the patient and he is reassured. An appropriate appliance for use following surgery is sent to the operating room with the patient. The use of an appliance in the operating room is important. It can be devastating to have the patient awaken following anesthesia and be bathed in stool, especially when the patient has been reassured prior to surgery that this is not likely to occur. The patient is seen by the enterostomal therapist in the recovery room.

The patient may be revolted by the stoma. As soon as he sees it, it is rejected. The patient may feel that it looks like a "lump of raw meat," and may be unable to look at it, stating that it is nauseating. They may hate the surgeon for giving them an ileostomy.

The enterostomal therapist can help the patient deal with these feelings. The patient is seen at least once a day. He may require from 30 minutes to four hours per day during the immediate postoperative period. The stoma is inspected daily, and measured in order to select a suitable appliance. There should be ⅛ inch margin around the stoma to allow for expansion. The pouches used in the immediate postoperative period are clear plastic so that the stoma can be observed without having to remove the appliance.

An unrestricted diet, unless medically contraindicated, is suggested. Patients are taught to chew their food well and drink lots of fluid with salt supplements. There are no foods which must be restricted.

The patient is encouraged to have an ostomy visitor before and after surgery. Patients can often benefit significantly from such a visit. They can identify with their visitor and see him as someone who has recovered and is now leading a normal life. The new ostomate can see that the ostomy visitor can work full time and not live in dread that he is continuously exposed to some horrible disease. The patient can be reassured that an adjustment to a normal lifestyle is likely and should be anticipated.

Many appliances are available today. Figure 30-2 shows a Hollister appliance. It has microporous adhesive around a karaya seal, which is open and drainable. The seal generally lasts two to three days. Some patients can wear it as long as five days. They are odor-proof. The patient is taught to empty the pouch four to six times a day, and encouraged to rinse it out once or twice a day and before they retire at night. Occasionally an odor problem will require individual management, but this can be corrected.

Figure 30-3 shows a Stomahesive with a Coloplast pouch. A Reliaseal disc can also be used. This appliance can remain in place for seven to ten days. The Reliaseal tends to be more durable than the karaya washer in hot climates. It has a double-faced adhesive. One side is blue and the other side, which is applied to the skin, is white.

Figure 30-4 shows a Grier one-piece reusable appliance which is applied with a Collyseal. This Collyseal is modified karaya which makes it more durable. This would require changing of the appliance every four to seven days. The pouch is reusable, following cleaning, for up to three to four months.

The Hollister appliance costs approximately $26.00 for a box of 30, or about $265.00 a year. Use of adjunctive materials can increase the annual cost from $300 to $1200 a year, depending upon how often the appliance is changed.

Congress passed a law in September 1976 making ostomy equipment tax-free. The patient should be advised of this. Medicare will pay 80% of the cost of the appliances after the annual deductible has been met. Medicaid, likewise, will pay for the appliances. Some insurance companies will also provide for stoma care.

The fees of enterostomal therapists are not covered by insurance policies. The hospital provides a service for inpatients. Outpatients are unable to be reimbursed, however.

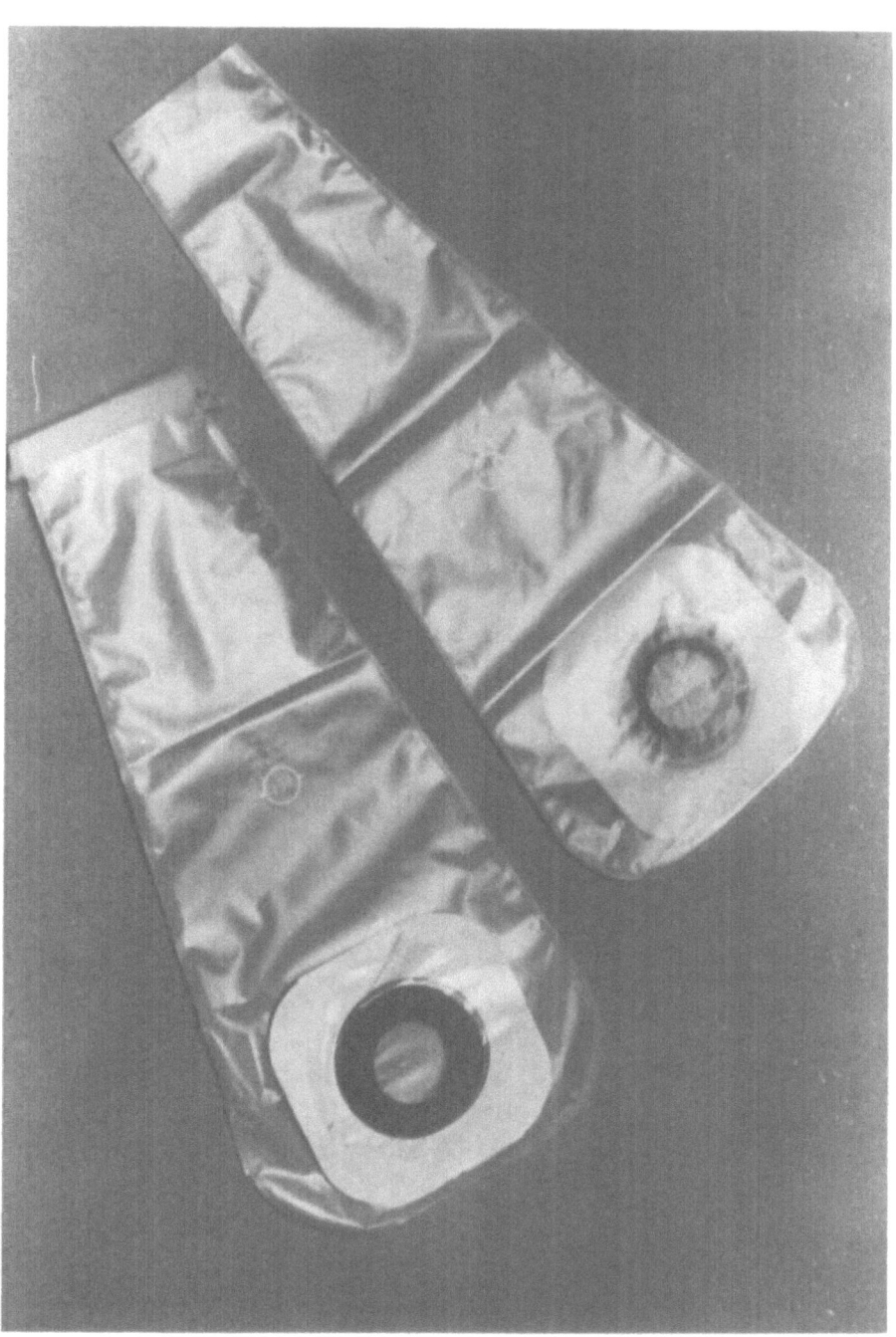

Figure 30-2 Hollister appliance.

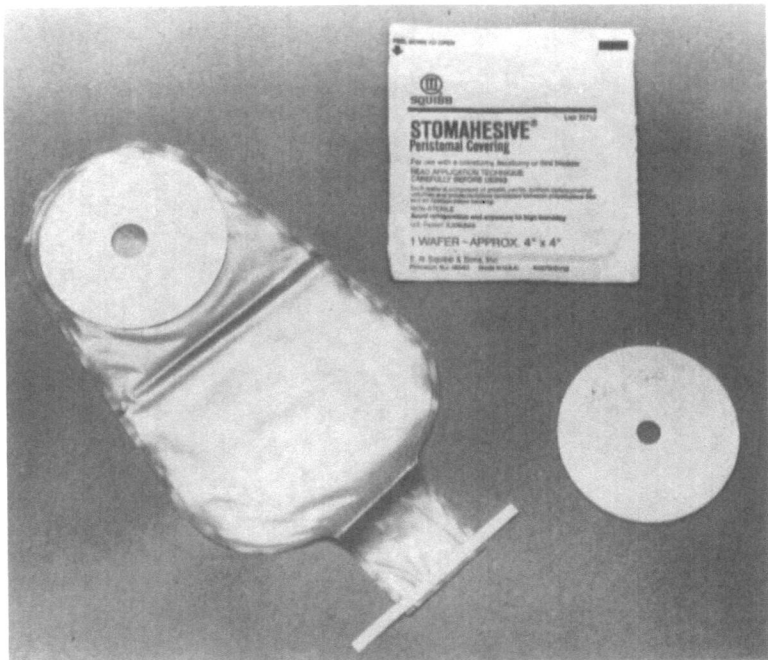

Figure 30-3 Stomahesive (peristomal covering).

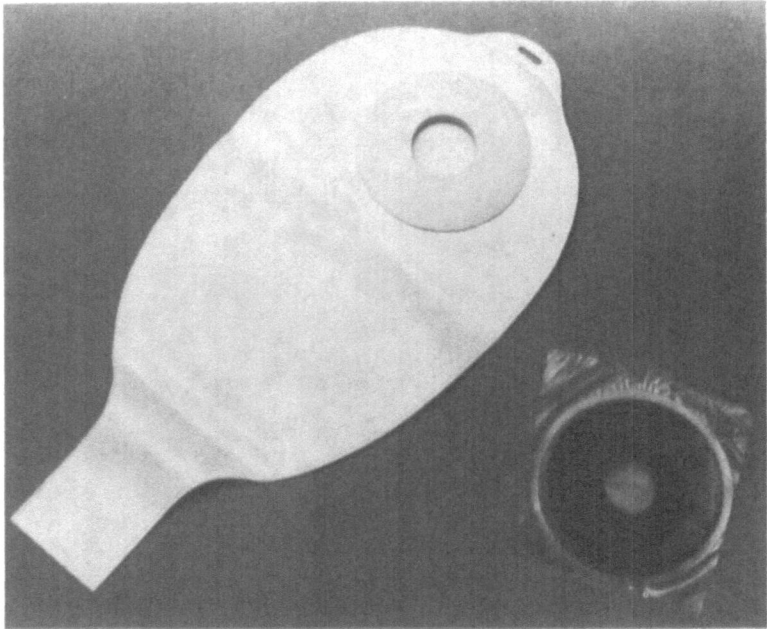

Figure 30-4 Grier one-piece, reusable appliance.

Clothing should present no problem. The patient should be able to wear what he has been accustomed to wearing in the past. A well-created stoma with a neatly fitting appliance which is nonbulky and associated with good hygiene necessitates very little modification of the patient's clothing.

Patients are encouraged not to use gloves when changing their appliance. This suggests rejection of the stoma. Nor should the therapist use gloves when providing stomal care, unless there are abrasions of the skin, or if the patient is on skin and wound precautions. Changing the appliance should be treated as a normal procedure. Just as gloves were not used following bathroom functions prior to the operation, they should not be used following surgery.

The patients are advised to associate themselves with an Ileostomy Club. This enables them to socialize with people who have met their problems previously and are engaging in various techniques for coping with these problems. It provides them with education and up-to-date information on the care of stomas.

Physician follow-up is also important. The therapist sees the patient approximately six weeks following discharge and again at 12 weeks, six months, and annually thereafter. The stoma should be recalibrated at these visits. Modifications as to the type and selection of appliance may have to be made. This is certainly the case if the patient has gained weight. These visits are also used to educate the patient in the prevention and management of stoma-related complications.

Home care, family counseling, and vocational rehabilitation resources can be made available to the patient on an individual basis.

BIBLIOGRAPHY

Goldblatt M: Ileostomy complications requiring revision. *Dis Colon Rectum* 20:209–214, 1977.

Phipps CL: Physicians have them too. *Ostomy Quarterly*. Fall, 1978.

Rogers G: Complications of ileostomy life. *Ostomy Quarterly* Spring, 1977.

Steiger B: *My Ostomy and Yours*. Chicago, Hollister Inc, 1976.

Turnbull B Jr, Weakley F: Ileostomy. *Crafts of Surgery*. Boston, Little, Brown & Company, 1974, pp 1141–1148.

Turnbull G: A portrait of the inflammatory bowel disease patient. *ET Journal*, Vol 5, No 4, Fall 1978.

31 The Continent (Kock) Ileal Reservoir: Technique and Indications

Felicien M. Steichen, MD

Following total proctocolectomy for ulcerative colitis, ileostomy either of the conventional type or the continent type (Kock reservoir) is required. In order to better understand what the construction of a continent ileostomy and reservoir entails, the technique of the Kock pouch is briefly reviewed.

TECHNIQUE OF CONTINENT ILEOSTOMY AND RESERVOIR

The construction of a Kock pouch is started by delineating its various component parts. The efferent loop of the reservoir, leading to the ileal stoma, should measure at least 10 cm, with the projected nipple situated at 5 cm from the pouch or reservoir itself. Proximal to the efferent loop, 30 cm of ileum are measured and folded in a U-shaped fashion at the 15-cm mark, so as to obtain two parallel 15-cm segments. By joining the apposing sides of these loops with a suture and then incising the antimesenteric vortex of the bowel anterior to this suture line, a flat, racquet-shaped segment of bowel is obtained. This step of the procedure can be greatly facilitated by the use of special mechanical suture instruments as shown in Figure 31-1A and B. The instrument shown here places four lines of hemostatic staples in successive applications, using a special mechanical suture or staple cartridge. The bowel walls are incised anterior to the instrument, with the instrument in place used as a guide for these incisions.

Following this first step, the nipple assuring continence is constructed. As a preliminary step to the nipple construction, the mesentery at the site of the nipple is excised and denuded in order to diminish the bulk of the mesentery as it is intussuscepted together with the bowel wall. A special suture is placed in order to facilitate the rotation of the mesentery (Figure 31-1C).

As the intussusception progresses and the future nipple takes shape, the special suture on the outside wall of the bowel is tied as seen in Figure 31-1D. Later, other sutures are taken from the outside wall of the base of the nipple to the outside wall of the remaining efferent loop in order to maintain the nipple in place. In addition to the out-

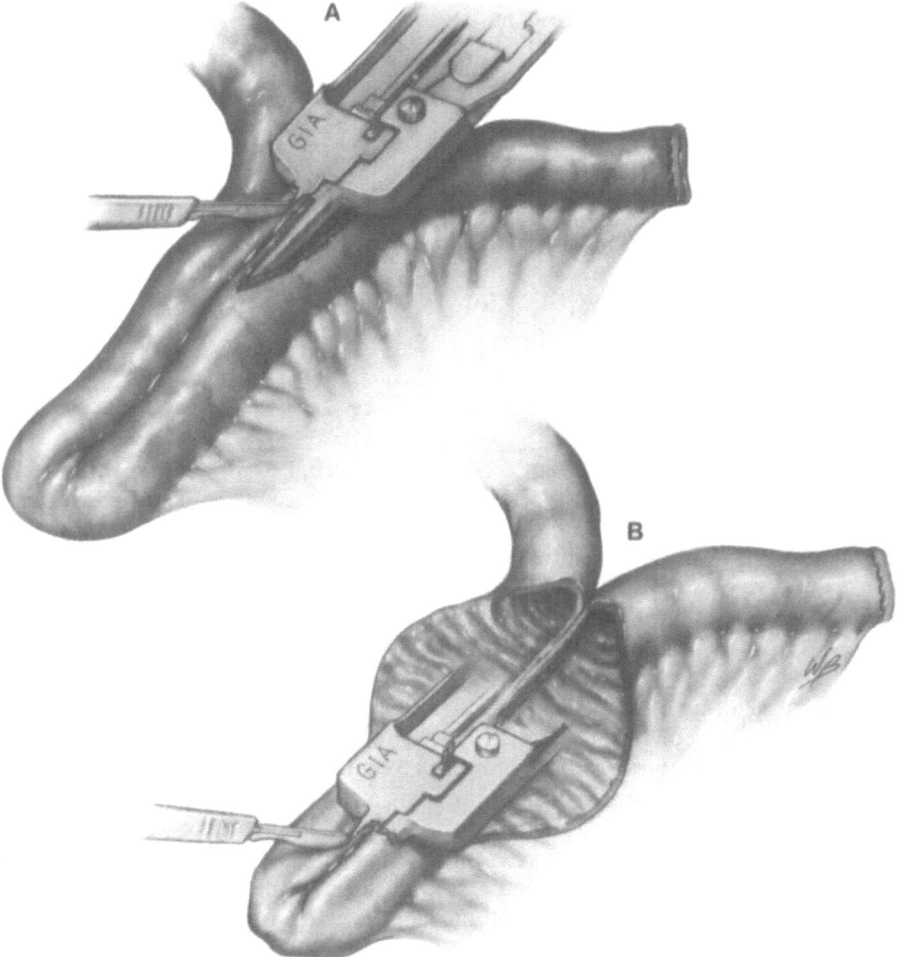

Figure 31-1A, B Stages in construction of continent (Kock) ileostomy and reservoir.

side sutures, the nipple, having a strong tendency to dislocate in order for the bowel to return to its normal position, is maintained with the application of three to four rows of mechanical sutures placed at two, five, eight and eleven o'clock, again using a special staple or mechanical suture cartridge (Figure 31-1E). At the end of this procedure the nipple should clearly project into the future reservoir.

At this point the construction of the future pouch is continued by folding the racquet-shaped bowel segment at its midportion along a transverse axis. The closure of the reservoir is then completed by either mechanical or manual sutures as shown in Figure 31-1F and G. If manual sutures are used, they are placed in a double layer fashion.

Bowel function is then examined by inserting a catheter into the reservoir and injecting saline and air while the afferent ileal loop is clamped. The catheter should move with

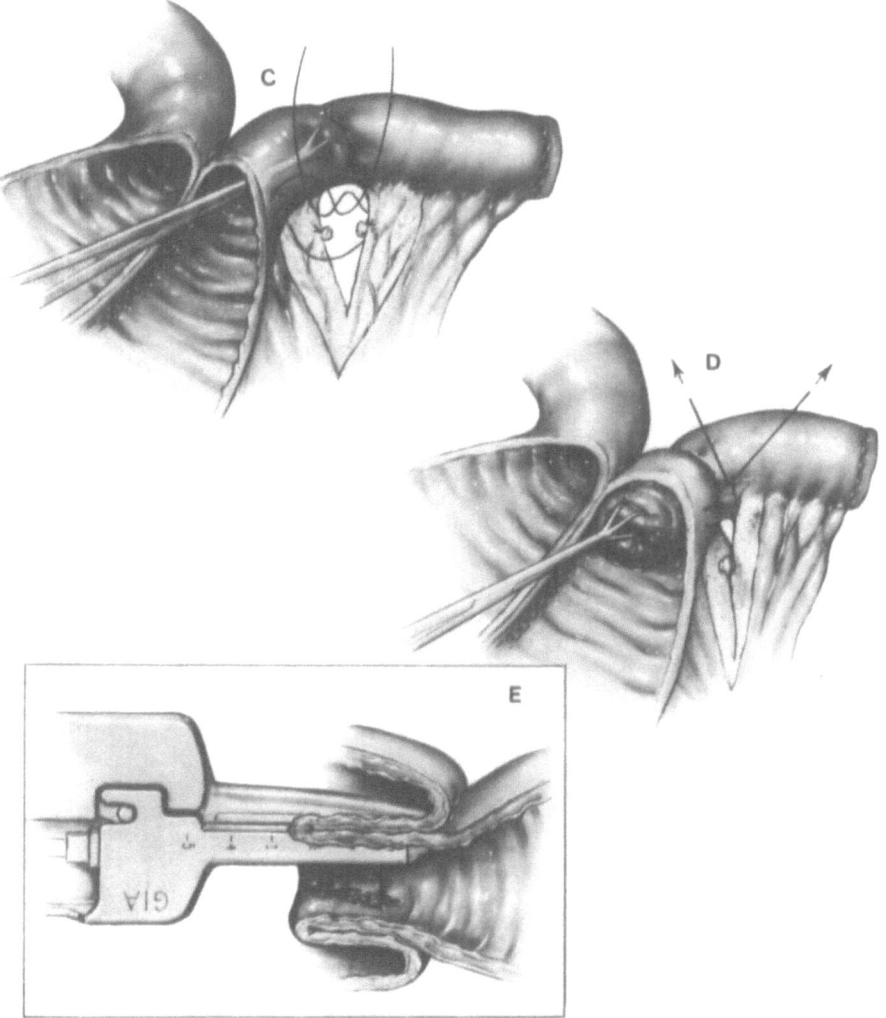

Figure 31-1C, D, E Stages in construction of continent (Kock) ileostomy and reservoir.

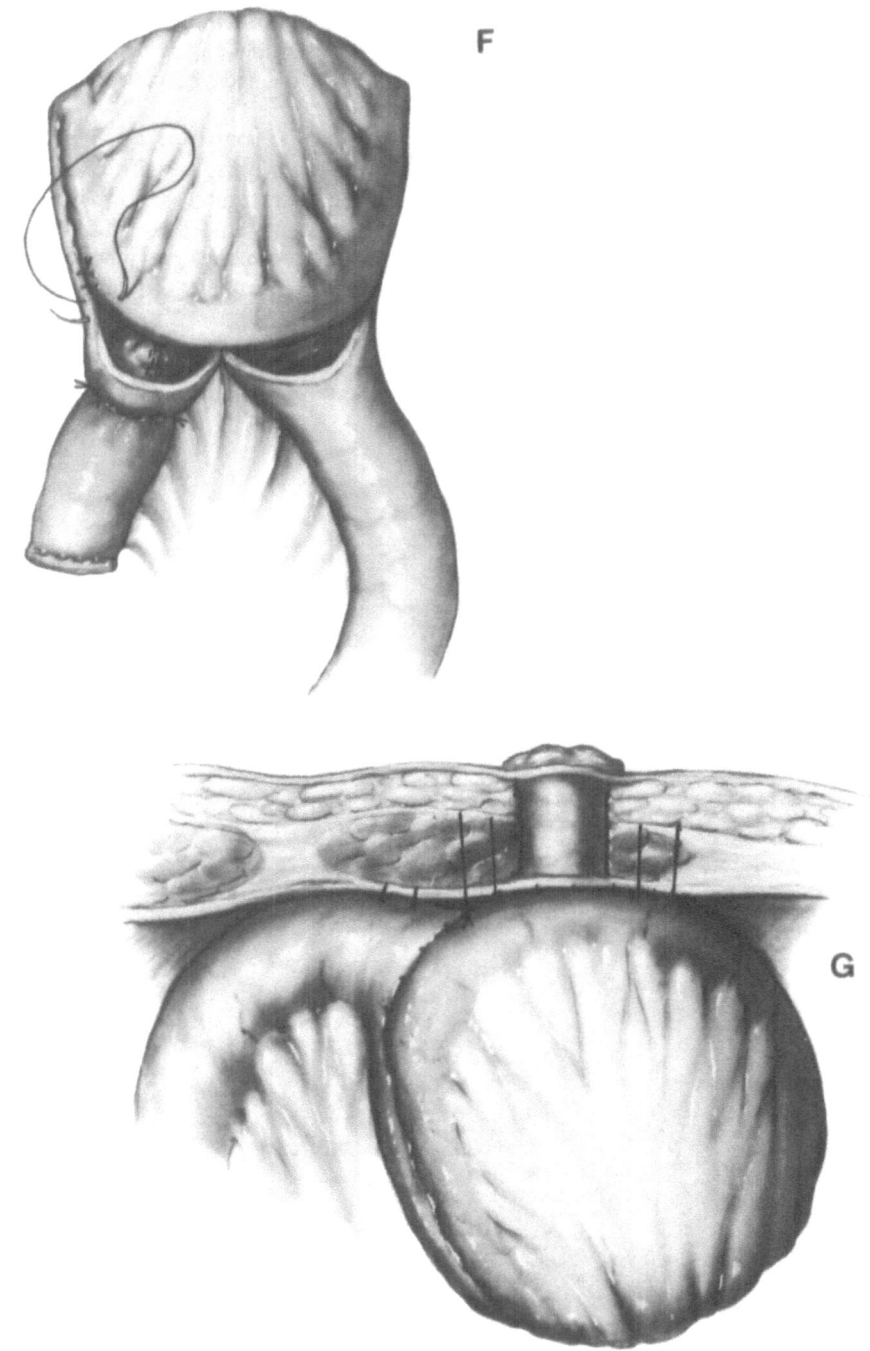

F

G

Figure 31-1F, G Stages in construction of continent (Kock) ileostomy and reservoir.

ease through the nipple and there should be no leakage of air or water through the outlet after the catheter has been removed. The reservoir is evacuated by reinserting the catheter.

As a final step the reservoir is placed into the pelvis, and the stoma on the abdominal wall is created in a fashion that permits the patient to introduce the catheter with great ease. On thin patients, for instance, this should be low enough so that they can wear a normal bathing suit. The straight channel created through the abdominal wall for the placement of the stoma is at the lateral border of the right rectus muscle and penetrates through the lateral fibers of this muscle.

Much of the success of this operation is due to very careful postoperative attention to many details directed essentially at removing bowel contents from the pouch continuously and avoiding any pressures on the nipple. Indeed, some surgeons do recommend a proximal temporary ileostomy in order to give the pouch a chance to heal without any pressures or actions by the bowel contents. In our personal experience we have used an indwelling ileostomy catheter and have maintained this in position for a three-week period. During these three weeks the catheter is cleared several times a day with 15 ml to 20 ml of saline and connected to straight drainage. As bowel activity returns, nasogastric suction and intravenous fluids are discontinued in approximately five to six days after operation, and the patient starts on a progressively increasing diet both in consistency and in calories. After the three-week period of straight drainage has elapsed, intermittent catheter drainage of the reservoir is started, first by emptying the pouch every two hours during the day and leaving it on straight drainage during the night another two to three weeks. Then, very progressively, the time between drainage is increased, first during the day and later at night, to a six- to eight-hour tolerance.

As a brief review of the various technical details demonstrates, even to the non-surgeon, the creation of a continent ileostomy is much more involved than that of a conventional or Brook's ileostomy. Therefore, in addition to considering the advantages and disadvantages of both procedures, physicians and surgeons interested in the operative treatment of a given patient have to consider and respect the various facts that may enter into the decision making.

INDICATIONS FOR CONVENTIONAL ILEOSTOMY

In Crohn's colitis, conventional ileostomy is absolutely indicated. While the surgeon does have a choice in ulcerative colitis, the continent ileostomy should never be used in a patient with Crohn's colitis for fear that the small bowel used in the creation of the reservoir may be involved with the same disease process. Similarly, if the pathological diagnosis after preliminary biopsy is questionable in patients where the clinical evolution is not helpful to make a differential diagnosis between Crohn's disease and ulcerative colitis, then a conventional ileostomy should be used each time, at least as a preliminary step. Finally, in patients who have undergone malignant transformation of ulcerative colitis, conventional ileostomy is preferred in order to see the long-term evolution of the patient, perhaps reserving the reservoir for a later period as the patient weathers the test of time (Tables 31-1 and 31-2).

The general condition of a given patient may influence the choice of operation since the creation of the conventional ileostomy adds very little to the overall operation, whereas the construction of a continent ileal pouch almost doubles the operating time and adds to the potential morbidity of the operation. The judgment as to the choice of

Table 31-1
Conventional Ileostomy Indications

Crohn's diagnosis	No experience continent ileostomy
Questionable diagnosis	Patient physiology
Malignancy	Poor general condition
Single-stage operation	Preoperative steroids

Table 31-2
Conventional Ileostomy Advantages and Disadvantages

Advantages	Disadvantages
Easy to construct	Unsightly eversion
Test of time	Incontinence
No intrinsic mortality	Appliance
Minimal morbidity	Odor
Revision rate 2%	Skin irritation
Long-term adaptation	Fluid, sodium loss
	Bile acids malabsorption
	Vitamin B_{12} malabsorption
	Quality of life 50%

operation does require experience with both procedures, especially in patients who have had cardiovascular, pulmonary, or renal problems, or who are in generally poor nutritional state, or who have been on prolonged preoperative steroids. All these conditions would favor the use of a conventional ileostomy.

INDICATIONS FOR CONTINENT ILEOSTOMY

A continent ileostomy can be used in patients with ulcerative colitis and familial polyposis. As surgeons acquire more experience with this approach, it becomes apparent that not every patient will do well with a continent ileostomy, nor even accept the need for intubating and draining the reservoir several times a day. Therefore, there has to be patient selection, based on experience and a certain anticipation as to the type of patient who will do well with a continent ileostomy. The patient has to demonstrate a strong motivation after all of the intricate details of the continent ileostomy have been explained, and the cooperation between the surgeon and the patient has to be an ideal one. Both must understand that there must be a total follow-up with easy access by the patient to an experienced surgeon who is able to cope with the various needs that arise after operation. Because of these special considerations, it is probably preferable to perform the colectomy and continent ileostomy in two stages. This will give the patient time to decide if he wishes a continent ileostomy based on his like or dislike of an incontinent, conventional ileostomy. In addition, it will avoid the rather lengthy one-stage colectomy and continent ileostomy operation (Tables 31-3 and 31-4).

Table 31-3
Continent Ileostomy Indications

Ulcerative colitis	Mutual cooperation
Familial polyposis	Second-stage operation
Strong patient motivation	Experienced surgeon

Table 31-4
Continent Ileostomy and Reservoir Advantages and Disadvantages

Advantages	Disadvantages
Skin level stoma	Difficult to construct
Continence	Added operative time
No odor	Morbidity, mortality
Clean skin	Vitamin B_{12} deficiency
Colonic physiology	Increase anaerobic organisms
Quality of life 80%	Revision rate 18% to 33%
	Need for cooperation
	Patient selection

COMMENTS

From a comparison of the various techniques, it is easy to conclude that the creation of a conventional ileostomy is technically simpler to accomplish and that this procedure has so far withstood the test of time. There is no intrinsic mortality related to the use of a conventional ileostomy in a given patient. The morbidity is minimal, requiring need for revision in only about 2% of patients. While patients with a conventional ileostomy lose water and salt, long-term adaptation by the patient to this condition is easily accomplished.

However, conventional ileostomy does require an unsightly eversion of ileal wall and mucosa. The bowel contents flow freely, requiring the wearing of an appliance with the occasional odor that can be embarrassing to the patient and his surroundings. If the construction of the ileostomy is not perfect and if the fitting of the collecting appliance is not equally so, there will be a skin irritation which can be quite bothersome to the patient. In addition to the chronic fluid and salt loss, studies have shown that these patients suffer from malabsorption of bile acids and vitamin B_{12}, although this is usually asymptomatic. These factors can obviously be supplied orally to the patient and, if he is correctly coached, he can also compensate for fluid losses when traveling in warm climates or suffering from diarrhea.

By contrast, the continent ileostomy and reservoir gives the patient a skin-level stoma, with continence and absence of any odors. If continence is absolute, the skin is clean. The mucosa of the reservoir develops a colonic physiology. The quality of life is satisfactory to the patient in 80% of instances, whereas this is true in only 50% of the patients having a conventional ileostomy.

However, continent ileostomy and reservoir are difficult to construct and add to the operative time if the procedure is performed in one stage with the proctocolectomy. If this is not the case, then a second operation with a second general anesthesia has to be undertaken. Because of these factors, there is a certain morbidity and possible mortality associated directly with the construction of the continent ileostomy, a procedure which is related essentially to the quality of life, not maintenance of life itself. Because of the development of a colonic physiology, there are increasing anaerobic organisms, and breakdown and deficiency of vitamin B_{12}. However, these substances can be substituted orally by the patient. Even in the hands of very expert surgeons, especially as they begin using this technique, there is a revision rate of 18% to 33%. Recognition of this factor as well as the need for a very careful postoperative follow-up both by the patient and the surgeon, requires intense cooperation between the patient and surgeon. Furthermore, some patients have not done well after they received a Kock continent ileostomy because of their refusal to accept the need for repeated intubation of the reservoir, drainage of the reservoir, and intelligent handling of ever-changing circumstances in the filling of the reservoir with gas and contents, depending on the patient's diet. Therefore, it is important for the surgeon to develop a screening technique by which patients who predictably will not do well with the use of Kock pouch can be eliminated. While psychiatrists can be helpful in this area, the surgeon must develop this skill on his own, since he is the only responsible judge in this matter and the only person to understand to what extent the patient will have to participate.

If a continent ileostomy is considered by both the patient and surgeon, a two-stage operation, performed at a time when the patient is off most drugs including cortisone, may have an advantage over a one-stage procedure. At such a time, the state of nutrition of the patient may be much improved as compared to the time he was a candidate for proctocolectomy. Finally, the addition of hyperalimentation has allowed us to prepare patients much better both for one-stage or two-stage operations.

In conclusion, the technique of creating a continent ileostomy and reservoir has been described and compared to the creation of a conventional ileostomy. The absolute indications of a conventional ileostomy and the relative indications of a continent ileostomy have been discussed. Advantages and disadvantages of both procedures are considered.

BIBLIOGRAPHY

Akovbiantz A, Lindenberg K, Robert N: Erfahrungen mit der Kontinenten Ileostomie. *Chirurg* 47:22, 1976.

Beahrs OH: Use of ideal reservoir following proctocolectomy. *Surg Gynecol Obstet* 141:363, 1975.

Gelernt IM, Bauer JJ: The reservoir ileostomy: Early experience with 54 patients. *Ann Surg* 185:197, 1977.

Goligher JC, Lintott D: Experience with 26 reservoir ileostomies. *Br J Surg* 62:893, 1975.

Kock NG: Intra-abdominal "reservoir" in patients with permanent ileostomy. *Arch Surg* 99:223, 1969.

Kock NG, Darle N, Hulten I: *Ileostomy, Current Problems in Surgery*. Chicago, Yearbook Medical Publishers, vol XIX, 1977.

Steichen FM: The creation of autologous substitute organs with stapling instruments. *Am J Surg* 134:659, 1977.

Steichen FM, Loubeau JM, Stremple JF: The continent ileal reservoir. *Surg Rounds,* September 1978, p 9.

Thow GB, Castro AF, Beahrs OH, et al: Present status of the continent ileostomy. *Dis Col Rect* 19:189, 1976.

Conventional Versus Continent Ileostomy, Editorial, *Lancet* 1:292, 1980.

32 Experience and Late Results with the Continent Ileostomy

Irwin M. Gelernt, MD

Many of the late problems seen in patients with ulcerative colitis could perhaps be avoided if it were possible to achieve an ideal ileostomy. Patients, their physicians, and their families would be a little less reluctant to resort to surgery. An ideal ileostomy should be easy to construct, be continent, ie, no appliance be worn, and must create no new diseases and problems.

TECHNIQUE

The procedure for performing the Kock reservoir ileostomy is the same when done as a secondary maneuver or in conjunction with a total proctocolectomy. The procedure is performed with the surgeon on the patient's left. A total of 40 cm of terminal ileum is used to create the reservoir, nipple valve, and outflow tract; 10 cm of the most terminal ileum (slightly more if there is a thick panniculus) are left untouched, to be used to form the valve and outflow tract. The remaining 30 cm of ileum are folded in a U-shaped pattern, with the outflow tract facing cephalad. The two 15-cm limbs are joined with a running absorbable suture along the antimesenteric borders (Figure 32-1A). The limbs of the ileum are then incised along the suture line, extending the incision 2 cm to 3 cm more proximally than the suture line on the afferent limb. This facilitates separation of the afferent (inflow) and efferent (outflow) limbs when the reservoir is closed. A second continuous absorbable suture is then used to approximate the two cut edges of the limbs to constitute an inner layer (Figure 32-1B). The most terminal portion of the ileum is then intussuscepted in a retrograde fashion to form a 3.5-cm to 4-cm nipple (Figure 32-1C).

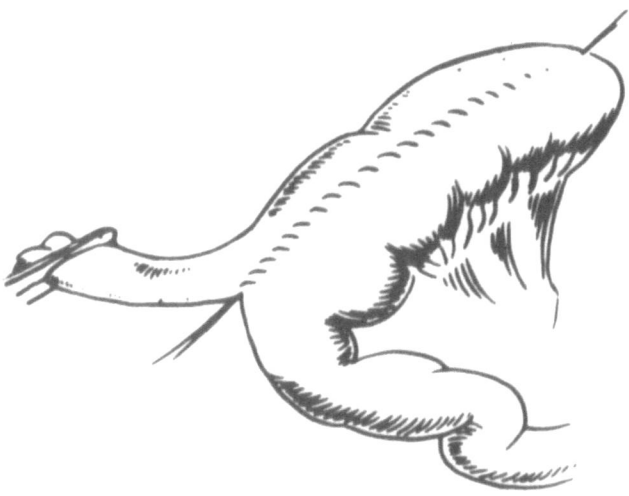

Figure 32-1A   The two 15-cm limbs are joined with a running absorbable suture along the antimesenteric borders.

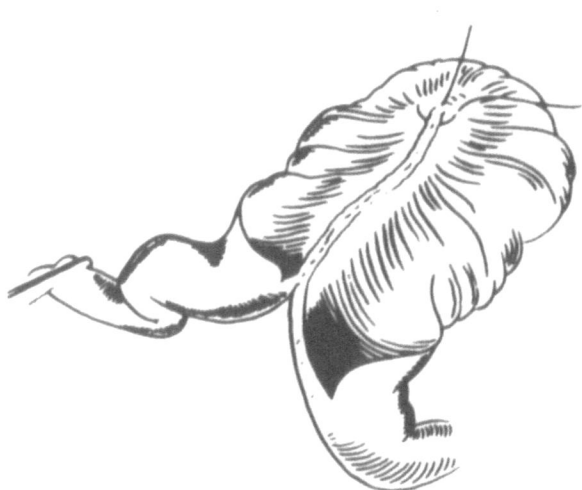

Figure 32-1B   A second continuous absorbable suture is used to approximate the two cut edges of the limbs to constitute an inner layer.

If the nipple intussuscepts easily, it is reduced, and the serosa of that portion of the ileum is abraded with a fine orthopedic rasp and scored with the cautery (Figure 32-1D). Two rows of four #2-0 seromuscular sutures are placed to plicate both mesenteric edges of the ileum (Figure 32-2A). When tied, the mesenteric edges of the ileum will have been fixed in a retrograde intussuscepted fashion (Figure 32-2B). The remainder of the intussusception is then performed, and a series of 12 to 16 #2-0 silk sutures are placed circumferentially perpendicular to the long axis of the nipple through both intestinal walls. A large-bore catheter or obturator should be placed in the nipple valve during suture placement to prevent inadvertent occlusion of the lumen by suturing the bowel of the opposite side. The sutures spare only the mesenteric aspect. The intestinal plate is closed apex-to-apex, as shown in Figure 32-2C with two layers of a running absorbable suture material (Figure 32-2D). The reservoir is folded into the leaves of the mesentery so that only the original suture line is visible. Valvular function is tested by occluding the inflow portion of the ileum, introducing a catheter into the reservoir, filling it with air, and removing the catheter. No air should escape when the catheter is removed.

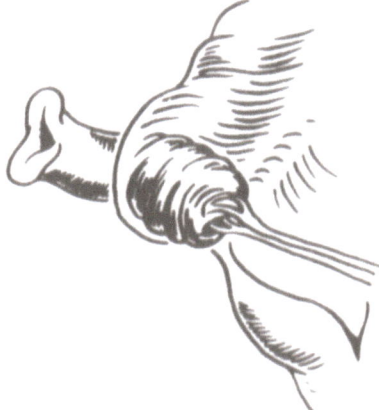

Figure 32-1C   The most terminal portion of the ileum is intussuscepted in a retrograde fashion to form a 3.5-cm to 4-cm nipple.

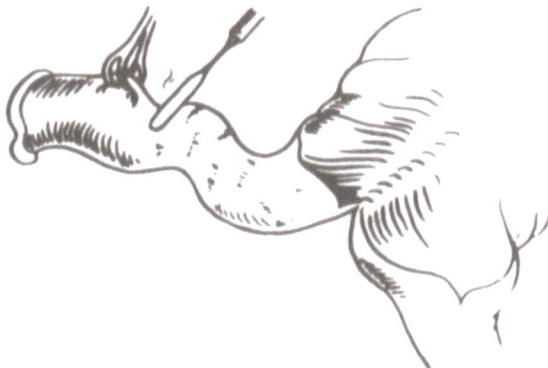

Figure 32-1D   If the nipple intussuscepts easily, it is reduced, and the serosa of that portion of the ileum is abraded with a fine orthopedic rasp and scored with the cautery.

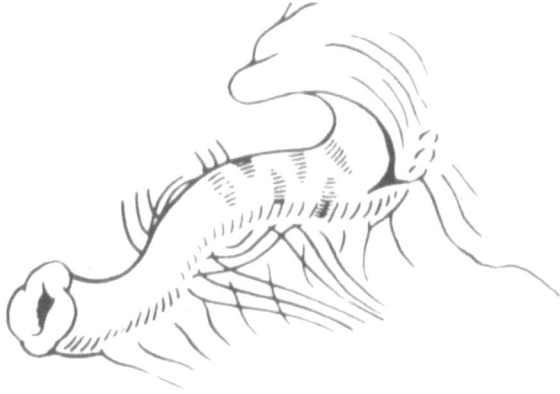

Figure 32-2A   Two rows of four #2-0 seromuscular sutures are placed to plicate both mesenteric edges of the ileum.

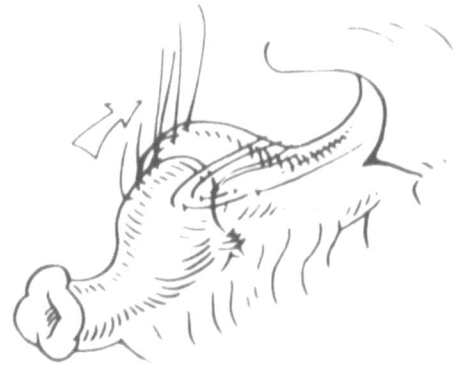

Figure 32-2B   When tied, the mesenteric edges of the ileum will have been fixed in a retrograde intussuscepted fashion.

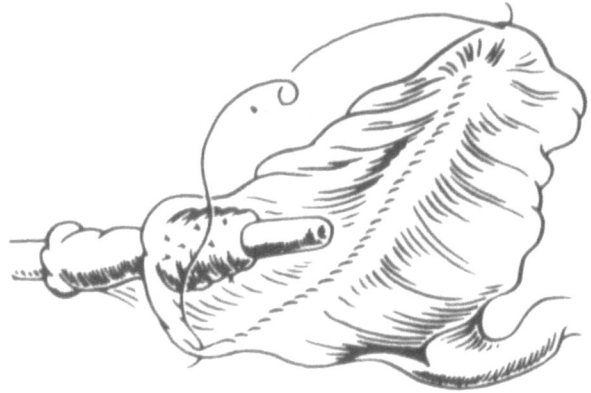

Figure 32-2 C The intestinal plate is closed apex-to-apex.

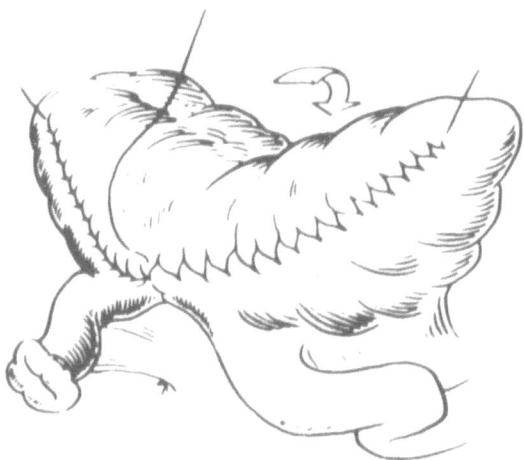

Figure 32-2D With two layers of a running absorbable suture material.

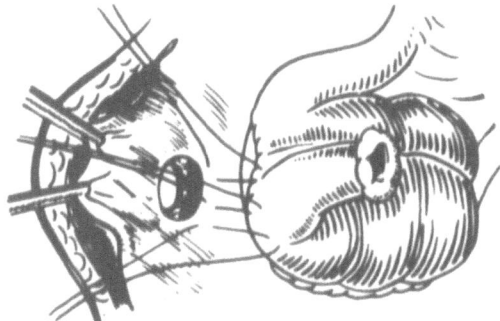

Figure 32-3A To facilitate proper fixation of the pouch, the posterior aspect of the reservoir immediately behind the outflow tract is fastened with silk sutures to the interior aspect of the peritoneal defect before the outflow tract is brought through the abdominal wall.

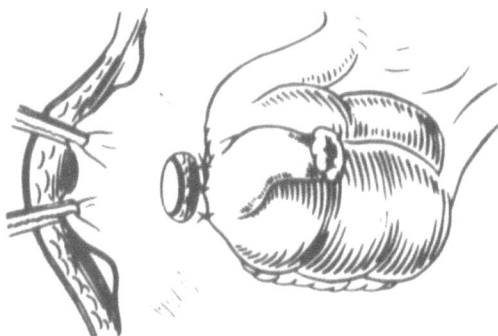

Figure 32-3B After the pouch has been securely fastened to the lateral parietes, the outflow tract is securely sutured to the abdominal wall with #2-0 silk.

The catheter is again introduced and the air released. A button of skin is excised in the right lower quadrant. The site is determined by choosing the area where the reservoir will fit best while resting on the pelvic peritoneum. The stoma will usually exist best just above the pubic hairline where it will be concealed by undergarments. A cruciate incision is made in the rectus fascia, and the muscle is divided bluntly in the direction of its fibers. An incision is made in the posterior fascia and peritoneum. To facilitate proper fixation of the pouch, the posterior aspect of the reservoir immediately behind the outflow tract is fastened with silk sutures to the interior aspect of the peritoneal defect before the outflow tract is brought through the abdominal wall (Figure 32-3A). After the pouch has been securely fastened to the lateral parieties (Figure 32-3B), the outflow tract is brought through the abdominal wall, and the remainder of the pouch about the outflow tract is securely sutured to the abdominal wall with #2-0 silk. The entire outflow tract must lie within the body wall. The outflow tract is amputated at skin level and the ileostomy catheter (A.B. Medina, Kungsbacka, Sweden, #28 Charriere) inserted into the pouch. It must traverse the canal easily and should be tested several times. The stoma is sutured flush at skin level, and the catheter is placed in the reservoir. It is important to confirm that the catheter is in a dependent position and that all of its openings lie within the pouch. The catheter is sutured securely to the skin (Figure 32-3C). Soft rubber drains are placed in the lateral gutter and exit via a lateral stab wound. The space lateral to the pouch is closed by suturing the mesentery of the ileum to the lateral parietal peritoneum. The ileostomy catheter is connected to a bedside bag via a wide-bore tube, and the wound is closed.

CONTRAINDICATIONS TO RESERVOIR ILEOSTOMY

There are a number of very definite contraindications to this procedure that must be strictly adhered to. There is no place for this procedure in patients undergoing emergency proctocolectomy, whether it be for toxic dilatation or hemorrhage. The additional 1 to 2

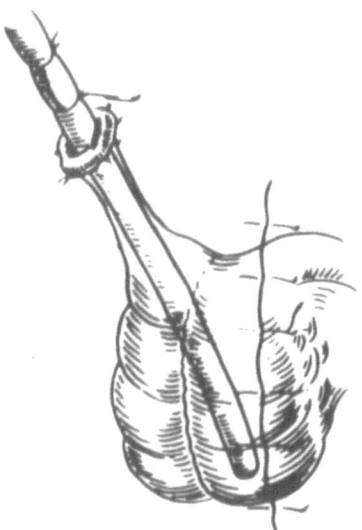

Figure 32-3C   The catheter is sutured securely to the skin.

hours of time spent in constructing the continent ileostomy is not justified in this situation. It would be much safer to construct the reservoir ileostomy at a second stage. If one studies the series described in the literature, it will be observed that the mortalities have frequently occurred in this setting.

We feel that this procedure is not justified at the present time in patients with Crohn's colitis. The incidence of complications in such patients was extremely high in Kock's series. It is well known that the recurrence rate of the transmural inflammatory process is considerable, and the risk for having to sacrifice 40 cm to 45 cm of terminal ileum is too great to justify the procedure in these patients. It is interesting to note that some of these patients have recurrences not only within the reservoir itself but also proximal to the reservoir, much the same as has been seen with procedures for Crohn's disease in which any anastomosis is performed.

Patients undergoing a subtotal colectomy should have a standard ileostomy. The presence of a reservoir in the pelvis would make it extremely difficult to remove the rectum in the future if it becomes necessary, as it almost certainly will. It is preferable to perform a standard ileostomy and, if the patient so desires, convert the ileostomy to a reservoir ileostomy at the time of removal of the rectum.

A cooperative reliable patient is paramount to achieving a successful result with this operation. The patient must be relied on to perform intubations in the proper manner, adhere to the rather rigid schedule outlined previously, and find it easy to insert a catheter into a new orifice located on the abdomen. Psychiatric complications of the Kock reservoir have been reported in patients who were not psychologically suitable for this type of procedure. We feel that the operation has no place in very young children because of the unreliability of such patients. It has been our practice, prior to accepting patients for the continent ileostomy, to spend considerable time in the initial preoperative interviews, explaining in detail the method used to empty the reservoir. We have the patient discuss the operative procedure and the postoperative management of the ileostomy with individuals who have had similar operations.

Finally, we feel that the procedure has a significantly higher failure rate in the markedly obese patient. Having seen many patients with poorly functioning reservoir ileostomies, which had been performed at other institutions, we believe there is a considerable higher valve-failure rate in the obese patient. This is undoubtedly due to the inability to maintain a proper retrograde intussusception when one is dealing with a very fat, thickened mesentery.

Why do results of this procedure differ in various centers? There is no question that if one adds an hour and a half to two hours to an already long procedure in a patient with severe debility or one who is having an emergency operation, there will be a significant number of complications, perhaps even death. Many errors have been made in the past. In patients who are subjected to subtotal colectomies and reservoir formation, it often becomes nearly impossible to remove the rectum and the reservoir becomes adherent to it. A number of surgeons here and abroad have had to remove reservoirs to get to the rectal segment. Many patients have had continent ileostomies created only following total colectomy. It is imperative that the pathological material be reviewed to make certain that the diagnosis is, in fact, ulcerative colitis.

EARLY POSTOPERATIVE MANAGEMENT

The catheter is left for gravity drainage for 14 days and is irrigated frequently to insure patency. On the 14th day, the catheter is corked for one-hour intervals and allowed to drain by gravity at night. The duration of corking of the catheter is gradually increased, and by the 20th postoperative day, the catheter is removed and the patient trained in its use. For several weeks, the patient empties the reservoir frequently, slowly increasing the times between emptying. Each patient is taught how to irrigate the pouch in the event this becomes necessary. In several months, the reservoir is emptied two to four times per day.

LATE POSTOPERATIVE MANAGEMENT

Immediately following construction, the reservoir volume is approximately 75 cc. The postoperative management is designed to allow the reservoir to increase slowly in volume so that there will not be a sudden build-up of pressure within the pouch, which cause a deintussusception of the nipple valve. Initially, the patient intubates the reservoir every two hours, gradually increasing this frequency by 30-minute intervals until the reservoir is emptied four times each day. At this point, the volume of the reservoir is approximately 500 cc. The patient will finally reach a regimen where intubation is necessary only two to three times per day. It must be stressed and reinforced with each patient that he should not go without intubation for too long a period. It has been our experience, in patients who had the reservoir ileostomy performed at other institutions, that too infrequent intubations too early in the postoperative period results in many patients developing nipple valve problems. The diet in the postoperative period is similar to that of patients with other types of bowel surgery in that they are initially started on a liquid diet and gradually reach a low-residue diet. We suggest that our patients have no fruits or vegetables for several weeks so that there will not be the problem of cellulose residue obstructing the catheter. Most patients return to an unrestricted diet. The patient with a continent ileostomy is aware that, if the stool becomes too thick, emptying will be prolonged; most patients have learned which liquids will help keep their effluent thin, so that emptying will be rapid. It has been our experience that grape or apple juice is quite effective in thinning stools; occasionally, the patient may require prune juice. On the average, a patient will spend approximately five minutes from start to finish in emptying the reservoir.

POSTOPERATIVE COMPLICATIONS

As with any major surgical procedure, especially a new one, there are many postoperative complications which may occur (Table 32-1). It is interesting that some of them have been reduced with increased experience; others, of course, cannot be reduced. Seven of our patients have had minor fecal fistulas. All have closed relatively rapidly with some drainage of the reservoir and all are now completely continent. Four patients have had major fecal fistulas at the drain sites. They could have been operated upon electively but they required a temporary loop ileostomy. Upon closure of the ileostomy, all patients have become continent.

This group has been significantly reduced in our second hundred patients, so that in choosing the right patient and the right situation to create a reservoir, one can avoid or reduce this complication. Fifteen patients have had intestinal obstruction or prolonged ileus. Five required surgical lysis of adhesions. These patients have now been followed

Table 32-1
Postoperative Complications in 200 Patients

Complication	No. of Patients	Comment
Minor fecal fistula	7	All closed rapidly with sump drainage of reservoir.
Major fecal fistula	4	Required temporary proximal loop ileostomy. All fistulae closed.
Intestinal obstruction or or prolonged ileus	15	5 patients required surgical lysis of adhesions.
Hemorrhage from reservoir	9	4 patients required transfusion.
Pulmonary embolus	2	
Bleeding or perforated gastric ulcer	2	Both received large doses of steroids. One had intestinal obstruction.
Skin stricture	6	Minor procedure with 36 hrs of hospitalization.

for seven years. The statistics are similar to those reported in the literature for patients with total proctocolectomies and standard ileostomies. The incidence of postoperative obstruction from adhesive bands is very common in this procedure. We have had nine patients with bleeding from the reservoir. Four required transfusion. None required surgery. We have had two major pulmonary emboli. One patient died of a major pulmonary embolus on the 19th postoperative day. Two patients have had problems with peptic ulcer disease. Both had been given large doses of steroids. Midway through our experience, we became very confident of our ability to achieve continence, and so we became a little cavalier about placing the stoma beneath the skin level. These patients, as might have been predicted, developed skin strictions about the stoma, and we had to fix them with small Z-plasties, using local anesthesia and a one-night stay in the hospital.

If one obstructs the small bowel, stasis of bacteria within the reservoir may occur. It has been demonstrated that the bacterial count within a reservoir will be significantly higher than in patients with standard ileostomies. It never quite approaches the normal stool in number of anaerobes or colony counts, but it certainly does increase. A new syndrome has been reported in the literature related to the bacterial count in the reservoir, something which we have called pouchitis for want of a better term. Patients who go for long periods of time without emptying their reservoir early in the postoperative period, perhaps before there has been mucosal adaptation, develop a syndrome of watery diarrhea, occasionally with blood in the stool, elevated temperature, and weight loss. They have all the symptoms and signs of inflammatory bowel disease. However, the condition usually responds rapidly to treatment. The patient must empty the reservoir often, take a broad-spectrum antibiotic, and irrigate the reservoir for several days. If the condition persists, one must seriously question that the reservoir procedure has, in fact, been done on a patient with Crohn's disease. If the patient has been referred from another institution, do not accept only the pathology report. Have the slides reexamined by a pathologist experienced in differentiating ulcerative from granulomatous colitis.

Absorption in a reservoir ileostomy has not been a problem. The fecal weight of the reservoir and a standard ileostomy are essentially the same. The stool becomes a bit thicker as times goes on, with less frequent emptying. It never reaches the point where the stool becomes too difficult to remove from the ileostomy catheter. If it does, the patient need only increase his fluid intake, perhaps salt his food more heavily, or use some mild, natural cathartic such as grape or apple juice.

Phillipson's studies with d-xylose and protein absorption have shown that there has been very little difference between the reservoir and the incontinent ileostomy. A blind-loop–like syndrome will not occur if the patient empties at least twice daily. Vitamin B_{12} studies by Kock's group and others have demonstrated that this vitamin is well absorbed.

There is a natural concern about what the long-term results would be should the constant irritation and stasis become a problem. The mitotic index is being studied as a guide to possible future difficulties with neoplasia or other problems. Phillipson's studies revealed a brief early increase in mitoses which started to level off, and in the fourth and fifth year after surgery appeared to return to the control level.

The functional results after the initial operation in the first 100 patients are shown in Table 32-2. Ninety-two percent of our patients were continent; seven had minor fecal incontinence. This resulted in a few extra dressings rather than the small dressing that they were wearing, but this was not the kind of incontinence requiring a new appliance. One patient was incontinent and wore an appliance. He was subsequently reoperated upon and is now perfectly continent.

Table 32-2
Functional Results (After One Operation)

	No. of Patients
Completely continent	92
Minor fecal incontinence	7
Fecal incontinence (appliance needed)	1

As we increased our series to two hundred patients (Table 32-3), we still had only that one patient who was incontinent and wearing an applicance. Ninety-four percent of our patients were, in fact, completely continent. This is with a minimum follow-up of six months and a maximum of seven years.

Table 32-3
Continent Ileostomy: Functional Results in 200 Patients
After Initial Procedure

	Percentage
Completely continent	94
Minimally incontinent	5.5
Significantly incontinent (appliance needed)	0.5

Figure 32-4 shows a patient on the operating table. The skin incision is clearly visible. The patient, rather than wearing an appliance and having the stoma project about half an inch, is wearing a small Bandaid just above the pubic hairline, one easily covered by even scanty undergarments.

We have been fortunate in our first 200 patients in not having had to remove a reservoir. Such results can be achieved by proper patient choice. We have had one death from pulmonary embolus. We believe this was not related to the reservoir ileostomy. In our series of 200 patients, we have had to revise 17 nipple valves. Six of the patients were done because of incontinence, six patients because of difficult intubation, and five patients because of prolapse. All patients are now well and are continent.

The best way to demonstrate the anatomy in the late postoperative period is by flexible endoscopy. The endoscope is inserted through the stoma and nipple valve, a U-turn is made and the endoscope is advanced. The mucosa appears quite normal over the valve and the reservoir itself.

There are some nipple valve problems that can be resolved endoscopically. If minor incontinence exists because of an adhesion below the nipple valve and the side wall of the pouch, it can be cut with a catheter through the endoscope.

The problem of a pouch created in Crohn's colitis is a real one. Kock reported a recurrence rate of 30%. Figure 32-5 is an x-ray film showing recurrence in a patient with Crohn's disease. The recurrence was in the segment proximal to the reservoir, much the way it is with an anastomosis. We were fortunate in that we could just resect this segment and replug it into the reservoir which was normal both by biopsy and inspection. This patient is now getting along quite well. We are, of course, awaiting his next recurrence and the possibility of having to sacrifice the reservoir.

In summary, we believe that the continent ileostomy has been an advance in the treatment of ulcerative colitis and the familial polypsis syndrome. The procedure has now progressed beyond the experimental stage. It is a more readily acceptable alternative for the patient requiring colectomy than the better-known protruding ileostomy.

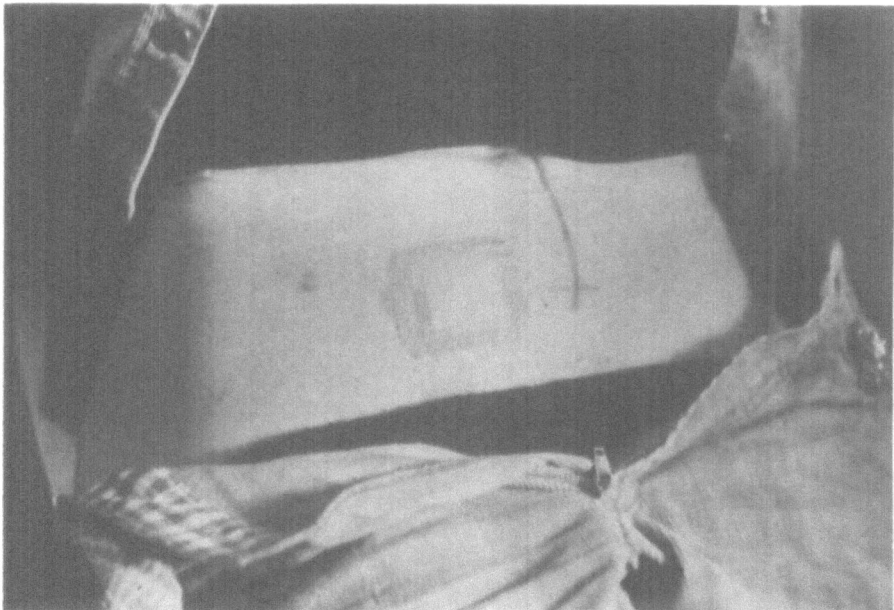

Figure 32-4 This figure shows a patient on the operating table. The skin incision is clearly visible.

218

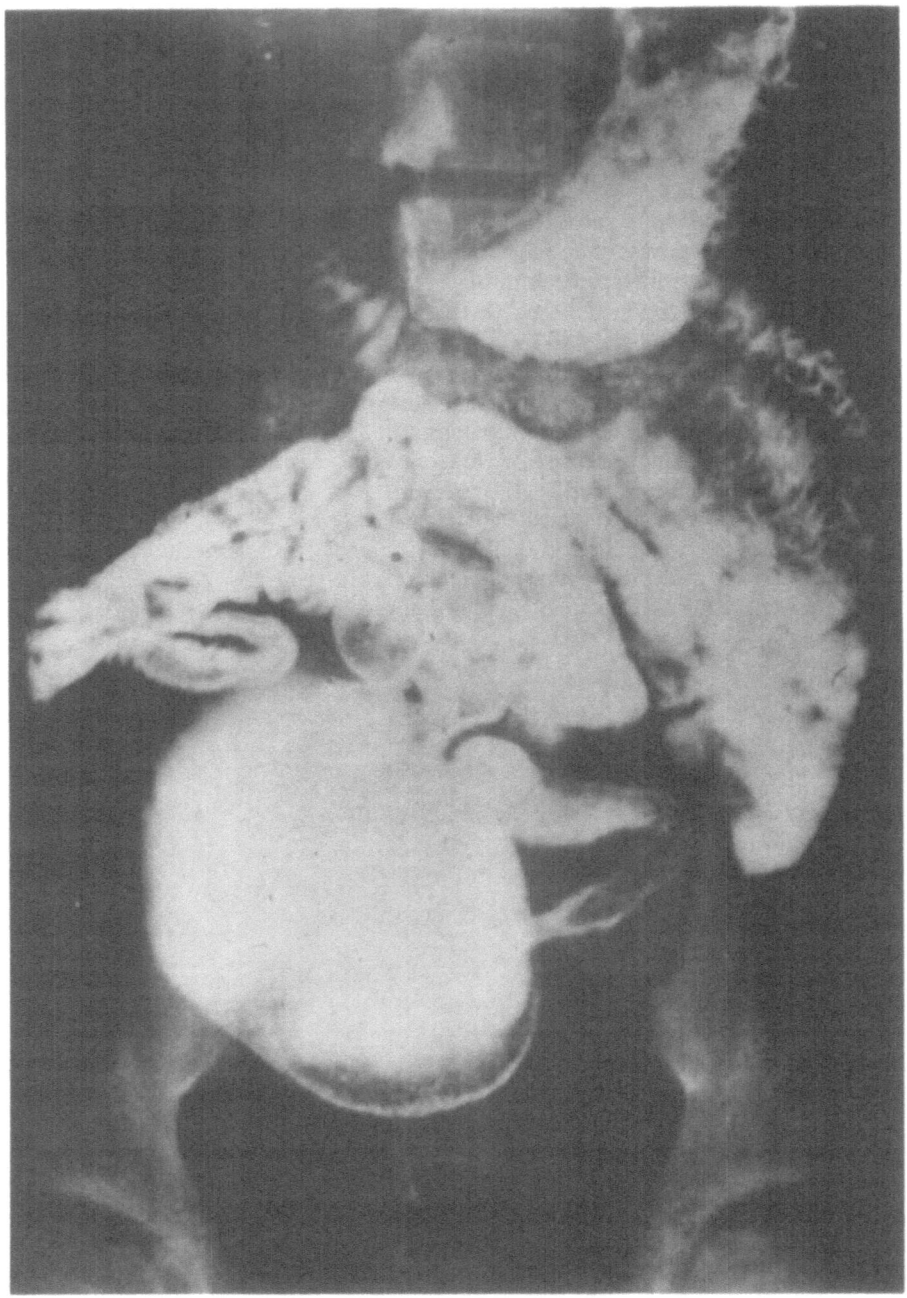

Figure 32-5 This x-ray shows recurrence in a patient with Crohn's disease.

BIBLIOGRAPHY

Branberg A, Kock NG, Phillipson B: Bacterial flora in intraabdominal ileostomy reservoir. *Gastroenterology* 63:413, 1972.

Gelernt IM, Bauer JJ, Kreel I: Early experiences with 54 patients. *Ann Surg* 185:197, 1977.

Gelernt IM, Bauer JJ, Kreel I: The continent ileostomy. *Practical Gastroenterology* 1:47, 1977.

Goldman SL, Rombeau JL: The continent ileostomy. *Dis Colon Rectum* 19:192, 1976.

Kock NG: Ileostomy without external appliance: A survey of 25 patients provided with intra-abdominal intestinal reservoir. *Ann Surg* 173:545, 1971.

Kock NG, et al: *Ileostomy in Current Problems in Surgery.* Chicago, Yearbook Medical Publishers, vol XIX, 1977.

Kock NG, Darle N, Dewenter J, et al: The quality of life after proctocolectomy and ileostomy: A study of patients with conventional ileostomies converted to continent ileostomies. *Dis Colon Rectum* 17:287, 1974.

Phillipson B, Brandberg A, Jagenberg R, et al: Mucosal morphology, bacteriology and absorption in intraabdominal ileostomy reservoir. *Scand J Gastroenterol* 10:145, 1975.

Phillipson B, Kock NG, Robinson WL, et al: Function and stricture of the mucosa of continent ileostomy reservoir in dogs. *Gut* 16:132, 1975.

Waye JD, Gelernt IM: Endoscopy of the continent ileostomy. *Gastrointest Endosc* 23:196–198, 1977.

33 An Appraisal of the Results of the Continent Ileostomy (As Seen by the Gastroenterologist)

Daniel H. Present, MD

Why should we even try to consider subjecting patients to continent ileostomies? We have learned that most conventional ileostomates lead full lives. They are rehabilitated, most work full time, rarely is there any need for dietary restrictions, and almost all function better after surgery than when they were ill. They have increased earnings, participate fully in athletics (swimming, jogging) and bear children. Why, then, are we considering a new technique?

In any large series of conventional ileostomies, there are still a number of patients who are having difficulties, especially intermittent skin problems. This may be avoided with the help of a good enterostomal therapist, but many institutions do not have such therapists available. There may also be occasional cases of leakage, and other patients suffer with odor problems. There is some restriction in travel, and there are psychological reactions to the uncontrolled noise which may emanate from the stoma. There are sexual apprehensions, especially in those patients who have not yet established a normal sexual life prior to surgery (many of the young patients). In a recent sexual survey by Dr Brooke, 10% of married men and 14% of married women confirm that there are some sexual problems related to the ileostomy. Approximately 30% of patients reported that in some way the stoma was an embarrassment. Very few unmarried people responded to this survey, suggesting to the authors that they had a greater percentage of sexual problems, and were unwilling to discuss them.

Recently, Dr Kock and his associates presented an interesting group of ten patients who were felt to be functioning well with conventional ileostomies, and who were subsequently converted to pouches. They found that following conversion: ten out of ten felt they had increased confidence in themselves as individuals; eight out of ten noted leisure time was improved; working capacity was felt to be better in seven out of ten; sexual problems were somewhat diminished in four out of ten, although only one claimed that he had a better sexual life with the pouch; sports were performed better in three out of ten, and two out of ten had fewer problems with their clothing. Obviously, ileostomy function varies in different individuals, and only after conversion do some patients discover disadvantages of the conventional ileostomy. These conventional ileostomates did not note the above as major disadvantages before conversion, but it must be remembered that many of these patients had their conventional ileostomy because they were seriously ill. Compared to life with a diseased colon, the conventional ileostomy appeared to have a tremendous advantage, but only after comparison with the continent variety did the patients feel there was an improvement in the quality of their lives.

Although there are few surgical series reported, comparisons are not easily made. Kock's initial procedures were done without nipple valves. In addition to Kock's many modifications, Gelernt has added changes in the procedure. Thus it is difficult to review the literature and come to any valid conclusions. The mortality data reveals that Dr Kock, with the largest series of 277 patients, had a mortality rate of 2.5%; Beahrs' mortality rate was 1.3%; Gelernt's was 0.5%; Halvorsen's was 8.2%; and Goligher's was 0%. The reported continence was fairly good in all series; however, many of these patients required revision, and the initial continence data are often not reported. The excellent high continence rates of Kock and Beahrs followed only after numerous modifications and improvement of the nipple valves were made. The first 100 patients of Gelernt had a 92% continence rate.

With respect to the requirement for a second operation, Kock performed subsequent surgery in 60%. (Forty-two percent were nipple revisions, and the other 18% were necessitated by postoperative complications.) Subsequent surgeons taking advantage of the initial experience had lower reoperative rates: Halvorsen, 42%, Beahrs, 30%, and Gelernt, 10%. The continent ileostomy had to be removed with conversion to a standard ileostomy by Kock in almost 5%; Beahrs, 16%; Halvorsen, 17%; and Goligher, 23%. Gelernt's data have been the most impressive, and he has not had to take down any continent ileostomies. If all surgeons had Dr Gelernt's data of 94% continence, less than 10% reoperation rate, and a mortality of less than 1%, then this new procedure would certainly be considered for many other patients.

I have referred 12 patients to Dr Gelernt for surgery, all of whom are 100% continent, and have had a reoperation rate of 12%. The following are examples of typical patients sent for the continent ileostomy. The first patient was a 25-year-old female who had a 15-year history of ulcerative colitis, and was noted to have a stricture upon a routine barium enema surveillance. Colonoscopic biopsy showed atypia. Despite being completely asymptomatic and taking no medications, colectomy and ileostomy was recommended because of the stricture and atypia. The patient was reluctant to agree to surgery, but because of the internal pouch, accepted the procedure, and despite having a minor complication postoperatively (bleeding), has been totally asymptomatic and free of disease since the surgery. The second case was that of a 31-year-old male who had ulcerative colitis for 15 years which was controlled with immunosuppressives. Following discontinuation of the immunosuppressives on two occasions, the patient developed moderate exacerbations of his disease. Despite good control with this medication, surgery was recommended because of the protracted course of his colitis and possible increased cancer risk. The surgery was uneventful, and the patient did extremely well, is totally continent, and is not taking any medications.

What are the disadvantages to performing a pouch ileostomy? The multiple complications following surgery, both major and minor, have been discussed. There are also potential psychiatric problems. Dr Golden reported two patients who were converted from standard ileostomies to pouches, and then proceeded to mutilate themselves after surgery. He linked this procedure to a patient having cosmetic surgery. These patients were totally burdened with problems in their lives, had deep-seated dissatisfactions, and they felt that surgery would cure them of these problems. As Dr Gelernt has noted, these patients must be closely screened prior to surgery. Any patient who has had serious psychiatric problems, such as requiring ECT, who has been hospitalized for psychiatric problems, or who has taken psychotropic drugs for a protracted period must be closely evaluated before this procedure is performed. Perhaps one can anticipate whether a patient might be a candidate for the continent ileostomy by observing how he has handled his first operation.

As regards long-term complications, Dr Gelernt has previously mentioned pouchitis. Nonspecific pouchitis has been reported in 12% to 14% of patients and is characterized by increased ileostomy output, occasional bleeding, fever and weight loss. Pathologic findings in these pouches are nonspecific. Inflammatory changes are not usually seen in the small bowel above the pouch. This entity may be due to the increased numbers of Bacteroides and anaerobes in the pouch. Patients with this complication have responded to continuous drainage for a short time, and have also responded to Azulfidine (which does decrease total anaerobes). Other patients have been treated with systemic antibiotics and steroids. The pouchitis usually clears up in a few weeks, but occasionally may last a few months. Dr Kock has reported that he has not seen this in patients who have had the continent ileostomy for familial polyposis. This raises the question as to whether patients with inflammatory bowel disease are predisposed to this new illness. "Pouchitis" usually responds to therapy; however, we will have to follow these patients and see if there are going to be any long-term problems.

There is almost unanimous agreement among surgeons performing continent ileostomies that the procedure is not justified at this time in patients with Crohn's colitis. Dr Kock has created pouches in 37 patients with Crohn's disease. He reports one death and a 30% incidence of early complications. He has had to remove pouches in 11% of Crohn's patients, as compared to 3% of the ulcerative colitis group. In view of this high complication rate he also feels that Crohn's disease is a contraindication to a continent ileostomy; however, if you look at his initial group of 37 patients undergoing surgery, 26 are in excellent condition following the procedure. Therefore 70% of the total Crohn's group are doing well. Dr Korelitz has reported that Crohn's disease can be recurrent in a conventional ileostomy with a recurrence rate as high as 40% to 50%. Dr Gelernt recently performed a continent ileostomy on a 16-year-old patient of mine who was managed for 12 years with a typical picture of ulcerative colitis. This patient also responded to immunosuppressives, but because of chronicity and the high risk in a child of 16, I recommended an elective colectomy and continent ileostomy. The postoperative course was uneventful, but six months following surgery, he developed weight loss and fever. Barium studies demonstrated a six inch recurrence in the small bowel above the pouch. Retrospectively, this patient was felt to have had Crohn's disease rather than ulcerative colitis. We treated the patient with continuous drainage, Azulfidine and instillation of steroid enemas into the pouch. In 2 to 3 months he responded to treatment and has been in a total remission (taking no medications) with normal functioning of the continent pouch. This raises the serious question as to whether it is easier to treat recurrent Crohn's disease in a pouch *vs* recurrent Crohn's disease in a conventional ileostomy (with the latter you must often use systemic steroids with their high complication rate). It may be possible to treat these pouch patients simply with the instillation of medication. When this patient contracted his abdominal wall muscles, he could reflux the steroids into the involved small bowel above the pouch. Patients with ileitis in conventional ileostomies have increased fecal output and this output may be held back in a better manner by the pouch, and thereby result in better absorption of nutrients. I feel that a controlled trial in patients with Crohn's colitis is indicated. We could then monitor frequency of recurrences and the comparative difficulty of medical management. This controlled trial must obviously be initiated by a surgeon who has great experience with the procedure, and has a low morbidity and mortality rate in his ulcerative colitis patients.

How should a gastroenterologist view the continent ileostomy in terms of his patients with colitis? He must first have a surgeon with expertise in performing this procedure. Inexperienced surgeons should start with conversions from conventional ileostomies, rather than starting with patients who must undergo a total colectomy and a continent ileostomy at the same time. The gastroenterologist should refer patients who are having ileostomy dysfunction and/or chronic skin problems since this selected group of patients will need revision under any circumstance. The gastroenterologist should not "sell" this procedure to patients. If his patient is happy with the conventional ileostomy (as 90% to 95% are), the procedure should not be recommended. If the question of conversion is raised by a patient with a conventional ileostomy, the gastroenterologist must select those who are emotionally stable, who are well adjusted, and who have a desire for greater social and sexual freedom. He must then explain the potentially high complication rate, the prolonged hospitalization and the potential for a long period of being out of work or school. Strong contraindications are: immaturity in children; low intelligence; and psychological instability. Although it appears obvious to many, it should be reiterated that this procedure should never be performed in acute situations where colectomies are being done for bleeding, toxic megacolon, or sepsis. The procedure would be ill advised for a severely debilitated patient. I believe that Dr Gelernt has achieved excellent results because of his selectivity. He has refused many patients who have been sent to him for pouches, who are poor candidates for the above reasons. This firmness in not operating on poor risk patients is reflected in his low morbidity and mortality data.

In summary, my experience has been that continent ileostomy patients have been shown to gain self confidence, and have an improved quality of life. Gastroenterologists must first convince themselves of the effectiveness of the procedure, then carefully explain the complications, and finally, must allow the patient the option of making a final decision.

BIBLIOGRAPHY

Beahrs OH: Use of ileal reservoir following proctocolectomy. *Surg Gynecol Obstet* 141:363–366, 1975.

Gelernt IM, Bauer JJ, Kreel I: The reservoir ileostomy. *Ann Surg* 185:179–184, 1977.

Golden HK: Psychiatric casualties following revision to the continent Kock ileostomy. *Am J Dig Dis* 21:969-973, 1976.

Goldman SL: The continent ileostomy: a collective review. *Dis Colon Rectum* 21:594-599, 1978.

Goligher JC, Lintott D: Experiences with 26 reservoir ileostomies. *Br J Surg* 62:893-900, 1975.

Halvorsen JF, Heimann P, Hoel R, et al: The continent reservoir ileostomy. *Surgery* 83:252-258, 1978.

Kock NG, Darle N, Kementer J, et al: The quality of life after proctocolectomy and ileostomy. *Dis Colon Rectum* 17:287-292, 1974.

Kock NG, Darle N, Hulten L: *Ileostomy, Current Problems in Surgery*. Chicago, Year Book Medical Publishers, 1977, vol xiv.

PANEL DISCUSSION

Dr Sohn: I wish to play the role of the devil's advocate and illustrate a case where many of the complications that can occur with a continent ileostomy have actually occurred.

In 1972 a 31-year-old male noted the onset of chronic ulcerative colitis. In January 1973 he had a panproctocolectomy and ileostomy performed in California for a toxic megacolon. He decided he wanted to try the continent ileostomy. He was not happy with the lifestyle the conventional ileostomy afforded him. In April 1975 he had a continent ileostomy. One week later he was reoperated for a lysis of adhesions which produced intestinal obstruction. He then did well until November 1975 when the pouch detached from the abdominal wall during a touch-football game. This resulted in a revision of the continent ileostomy because of difficulty in intubating the pouch. He did well for a few more months, but then developed incontinence which led to a revision in April 1976. In October 1976 he was again revised for incontinence and difficulty in intubating the pouch.

In January 1977 he had another revision for incontinence and three months later had still another revision for prolapse and nipple fistula. In January 1977 he again was incontinent. We first saw this patient a year later in consultation. The pouch was resected and a conventional ileostomy done. In August 1978 he had intestinal obstruction and again underwent a laparotomy. In March 1979 he was again obstructed, operated on, and postoperatively developed an intestinal fistula. This was treated with total parenteral nutrition and he was discharged from the hospital.

This is the type of patient who is considered for a continent ileostomy. He has probably become an intestinal cripple as a result of the efforts to improve his lifestyle.

I think Dr Present raised a very interesting question regarding the place of the continent ileostomy in Crohn's disease and I would like to question the panel about a hypothetical patient. The patient is 40 years old. Five years ago she underwent a panproctocolectomy and ileostomy for what was definitely Crohn's disease. She now has a flush stoma. Endoscopy of the stoma reveals no evidence of ileitis. Biopsies of the stoma are unremarkable. A gastrointestinal series and small bowel x-ray is absolutely normal. In summary, this patient had a conventional ileostomy done five years ago of Crohn's disease. There is no evidence of any Crohn's disease on current examination. She is on no medication. The patient requests a continent ileostomy. She is not satisfied with her current lifestyle. Dr Steichen, what are your comments?

Dr Steichen: I would send her to Dr Gelernt.

Dr Sohn: Dr Gelernt, I am sure you have seen patients like this. What would your approach be to this patient?

Dr Gelernt: We have categorically refused to operate on any patient where Crohn's disease was even suspected.

Dr Sohn: I will put the same question to Dr Present.

Dr Present: I would have Dr Gelernt perform the surgery as a controlled trial. This is a perfect example of a patient suitable for a trial if all the complications are explained to and understood by the patient. The fact is that this patient has a 50/50 chance of recurring anyway some time in her life. Since I am not a surgeon, it is easy for me to say "perform an operation," but I think if somebody does not try this we are never going to find out if this procedure is going to help Crohn's patients in the long term. I think that if the risks are explained, and the patient understands and is willing to undertake them the surgeon should be willing to undertake these risks for the patient. I predict that after ten such cases we will have a good idea as to whether to go further.

I also have great faith in the current medical management of Crohn's disease, especially since we have started using immunosuppressives. I predict that we will be able to treat these patients medically with sulfasalazine, antibiotics, steroids, and/or immunosuppressives, and keep them well. The one patient that I have so far, with recurrent Crohn's disease above a pouch, is doing well on no medication.

Dr Sohn: There is one problem. I think you were very lucky with that patient, in that the recurrence occurred in a segment that could be resected. The real problem with patients who have Crohn's disease and in whom you do a pouch is that, if they live long enough, almost all will have a recurrence. If this recurrence occurs in the pouch and it is such that a further operation is indicated, you have to sacrifice much more bowel than in a similar patient with recurrence in a normal segment of bowel, where you resect just 10 cm. Here, the total pouch must be sacrificed. This is what I would be very concerned about.

Dr Gelernt: We have many patients who have had multiple resections of small bowel for recurrent Crohn's disease, and I find that they do not become "bowel cripples" until they get down to 5 or 6 feet of bowel. Trying one pouch in a patient, even if it is later resected, would not cause him to become a bowel cripple. I certainly would not do a repeat pouch if there were recurrent problems that required surgical correction. There would be a loss of a foot and a half of bowel each time you do it.

Given the state of the art as we know it now, Crohn's disease should not be an indication for this operation. If a group of gastroenterologists and surgeons in an institution where surgery for Crohn's disease is being performed want to undertake a study with proper informed consent, proper protocols, and controls defined before the operation, in patients who are willing to be followed and who can be depended upon to agree to various kinds of medical therapy, it might be considered.

Question: Is there a problem with pregnancy and intubation?

Dr Gelernt: We have had three patients who have become pregnant and have had prolapse of their valves. Only one of this group of three has come to term, and the prolapse was no longer a problem. I am certain that when the patient becomes pregnant again, she probably will again prolapse. I do not think this is a contraindication to pregnancy since the prolapse can be easily repaired if necessary.

INDEX